Fast Track Surgery:
Trauma,
Orthopaedics and
the Subspecialties

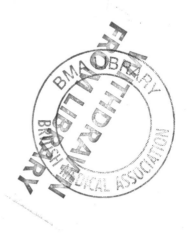

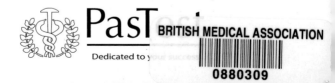

PasTest
Dedicated to your success

Also by Manoj Ramachandran:

Intercollegiate MRCS: An Aid to the Viva Examination (with Alex Malone and Christopher Chan) published by PasTest.

The Medical Miscellany (with Max Ronson) published by Hammersmith Press.

Clinical Cases and OSCEs in Surgery (with Adam Poole) published by Churchill Livingstone.

Coming soon from Manoj Ramachandran:

Basic Orthopaedic Sciences: The Stanmore Guide published by Hodde Arnold.

Also by Aaron Trinidade and Manoj Ramachandran:

Mnemonics in Surgery and *Fast Track Surgery: General, Vascular and Urology* both published by PasTest.

Fast Track Surgery: Trauma, Orthopaedics and the Subspecialties

by

Aaron Trinidade MBBS MRCS(Ed) DO-HNS
Senior House Officer in Otolaryngology, The Royal Free Hospital, London

and

Manoj Ramachandran BSc(Hons) MBBS(Hons)
MRCS(Eng) FRCS(Tr&Orth)
Paediatric and Young Adult Orthopaedic Fellow, Royal National
Orthopaedic Hospital Rotation, Stanmore, Middlesex

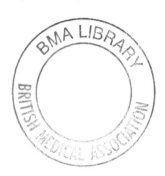

© 2006 PASTEST LTD
Egerton Court
Parkgate Estate
Knutsford
Cheshire
WA16 8DX

Telephone: 01565 752000

First published 2006

ISBN: 1 904627 95 1
ISBN: 978 1904627 951

A catalogue record for this book is available from the British Library.

The information contained within this book was obtained by the authors from reliable sources. However, while every effort has been made to ensure its accuracy, no responsibility for loss, damage or injury occasioned to any person acting or refraining from action as a result of information contained herein can be accepted by the publishers or authors.

PasTest Revision Books and Intensive Courses

PasTest has been established in the field of postgraduate medical education since 1972, providing revision books and intensive study courses for doctors preparing for their professional examinations.

Books and courses are available for the following specialties:

MRCGP, MRCP Parts 1 and 2, MRCPCH Parts 1 and 2, MRCPsych, MRCS, MRCOG Parts 1 and 2, DRCOG, DCH, FRCA, PLAB Parts 1 and 2.

For further details contact:

PasTest, Freepost, Knutsford, Cheshire WA16 7BR
Tel: 01565 752000   Fax: 01565 650264
www.pastest.co.uk   enquiries@pastest.co.uk

Text prepared by Type Study, Scarborough, North Yorkshire
Printed and bound in the UK by MPG Books Ltd., Bodmin, Cornwall

CONTENTS

ACKNOWLEDGEMENTS

As always, for my wife Joanna.

Manoj Ramachandran

Thanks again for the continuing support everyone has given me in this second of the series, in particular, my parents. Thanks also go out to Sandra Dieffenthaller who gave me a love of teaching. A special thanks to Kelly – your support was fantastic. Finally, thanks to Pastest for their patience during this project.

Aaron Trinidale

FOREWORD

Current surgical training is very structured, and requires junior surgeons to rapidly acquire knowledge and understanding of surgical practice, prior to progressing into higher surgical training. This is formalised in the MRCS exam. *Fast Track Surgery: Trauma, Orthopaedics and the Subspecialties* is an invaluable resource in achieving this aim. The book focuses on solid surgical principles with a structured approach to learning. This allows the junior surgeon to clearly appreciate essential points in patient care.

Broad knowledge, empathy and attention to detail are fundamental to the delivery of good patient care. Early in one's career, the required knowledge base may seem daunting. However a good understanding of basic surgical principles provides a solid foundation to care and facilitates further learning. This book highlights essential knowledge and provides a clear structured method of learning. This mirrors the teaching of basic surgical skills in the apprenticeship style training of good surgical technique. A solid foundation in both of these arms of surgery leads to the development of a competent surgeon. Moreover, it is this foundation that allows competent surgeons to develop into exceptional specialists.

More pressure is now placed upon the training process, to concentrate and condense this training. Attention and stress to structured learning, and the use of general principles and frameworks facilitates this process.

Ultimately the mark of a good surgeon is judgement, both in diagnosis and investigation, and particularly judgement in surgical care. This is the part of our profession that allows us to practise the art of surgery.

The authors of this book are enthusiastic, well motivated surgeons. It has been a pleasure to work with them. They have an excellent surgical understanding, and this is reflected in this clear, concise instructional book in surgical care.

It is a privilege to be a doctor and to be fundamental to care of our patients. With this comes a sincere responsibility to provide excellent surgical care. Personal improvement in provision of patient care is an ongoing task. This we all strive to achieve, through ongoing training, experience, study and research. This book provides a good foundation to understanding principles of care and facilitates the learning of the art of surgery.

Michael Papesch FRACS
Consultant ENT Surgeon
Whipps Cross University Hospital NHS Trust
Leytonstone, London

CONTRIBUTORS

Ravi Koka, FRCS(Ed)
Consultant Orthopaedic Surgeon, Eastborne District General Hospital, East Sussex

Chapter 5a   *General approach to management*
Chapter 5d   *Lower limb injuries*
Chapter 5e   *Tendinous, ligamentous and meniscal injuries*
Chapter 5f   *Compartment syndrome*

Daniel Horner, BSc MBBS
Senior House Officer in Surgery, Royal Albert Edward Infirmary, Wigan

Chapter 4   *The Trauma Call in Orthopaedics*

Daniel Tweedie, MA MB MRCS(Eng) DO-HNS
Specialist Registrar in Otolaryngology, London Deanery (South) Rotation

Chapter 8   *Otolaryngology and Head & Neck Surgery*

Dania Qatarneh, MA(Cantab) MBBChir
Senior House Officer in Ophthalmology, Queen Mary's Sidup NHS Trust, London

Chapter 9   *Ophthalmology*

Rhiannon Day-Thompson, MBBCh MRCS(Eng)
Senior House Officer in Plastic Surgery, Royal Gwent Hospital, South Wales

Chapter 10   *Plastic Surgery*

Swinda Esprit, BSc MBBS MRCS(Eng) DO-HNS
Senior House Officer in Otolaryngology, Wrexham Park Hospital, Slough

Chapter 11   *Neurosurgery*

Ibnauf Suliman, BSc(Hons) BM MRCS(Eng)
Senior House Officer in Cardiothoracic Surgery, Barts & The London Surgical Rotation

Chapter 12   *Cardiothoracic Surgery*

Jennifer Collins, BDS
Senior House Officer in Maxillofacial Surgery, Royal Sussex Country Hospital, London

Chapter 13   *Maxillofacial Surgery*

Amro Hassaan, MBBS DO-HNS
Senior House Officer in Otolaryngology, Charing Cross Hospital, London

Chapter 11   *Neurosurgery*

PART I

Introduction

CHAPTER 1: USING THIS BOOK

This book is a follow-on to *Fast Track Surgery: General, Vascular, and Urology*. It deals with the sub-specialist areas that you will touch upon during your time on the wards. Time spent in trauma & orthopaedics is much less than that in general surgery, and that spent in the other sub-specialties is even considerably less than that! Many students in fact view their time spent during these areas as a bit of a holiday and end up missing out on important clinical knowledge that would otherwise serve them well after graduation, only to lament later that the areas were never taught well while they were in medical school. The take-home message is this: your time in the sub-specialties is short but important, so make use of it; you'll be glad you did later on in your careers (especially if you do an A&E job or go into General Practice!).

The bulk of this book is geared towards Trauma & Orthopaedics, but the sub-specialties are each given their due. Only the most salient points and concepts are presented here, with focus being on the most-likely-to-be-asked questions. You are encouraged to read deeper into topics in standard textbooks and use this book as a study aid. By and large, as students, you are only expected to appreciate the basic concepts of the sub-specialties and have an idea of how to manage the common pathologies and emergencies.

As with *Fast Track Surgery: General, Vascular and Urology*, this book is laid out in a two-columned fashion to allow you to cover the answer column when revising. It leans heavily on mnemonics, tables and relevant in-theatre anatomy. Investigations and *the reasons they are ordered* are given, and management plans are laid out how you'd expect to see them written in the notes. Carry it around with you and cram from it in your precious spare moments.

When studying surgery, the following mnemonic is useful to keep in mind:

Dressed **I**n **A S**urgeon's **G**own, **A P**hysician **I**s **T**ruly **P**rogressing:
Definition
Incidence
Age Distribution
Sex
Geography
Aetiology
Presentation
Investigations
Treatment
Prognosis

This will form a framework on which to build your understanding of each case. The best way to learn is, of course, to clerk patients continuously, no matter how dull it may seem at times. Patients are a wealth of information. Following up the patient reveals investigations performed and management decisions made. This serves to bring to life what you've read and reinforces this information in your mind. But most of all, enjoy your time in surgery – medical school should be fun!

CHAPTER 2: SURVIVING TRAUMA, ORTHOPAEDICS & THE SUBSPECIALTIES

Depending on the sub-specialty, life on the wards can be pretty chilled out (eg otolaryngology) or can be really demanding (eg trauma & orthopaedics). Use the following tips to help you cope.

APPEARANCE

Dress smartly and make an effort to appear neat. You will see hundreds of patients, but the patients only see a few of you. White coats help, but be willing to take yours off if it makes a patient anxious (white coat hypertension). Remember you're on a ward dealing with patients, and not in a fashion show. Conservative is always better.

ATTITUDE

You *must* be a keener, but in measured amounts so as not to nauseate fellow students and junior doctors! Strike a balance. A lacklustre attitude leads to lacklustre teaching. Develop thick skin quickly. Sarcasm is common in surgery. Take things in your stride, not personally (unless it was meant to be personal). Be polite, especially to the ward sister who runs the show. Offer to do jobs. Speak up when spoken to, but never backchat. Humility is a virtue. If you can't be humble with your knowledge (or lack thereof), be confident with caution, but *never* cocky. Share information with colleagues and never show others up. Keep skiving to a minimum and make sure everyone pulls his or her weight: the adage 'one bad apple spoils the whole lot' rings true where most busy consultant surgeons are concerned, and you'll then have to really shine to avoid being grouped with slackers.

WHAT TO CARRY

Have the following handy at all times:

- Notebook and pen (have one extra for junior doctors)
- Stethoscope
- Tongue depressors (while in ENT)
- Penlight (handy for lumps and bumps and looking in throats)
- Blood and X-ray forms
- This book!

FIRST THING IN THE MORNING, DON'T LOITER!

- Make sure you're there first and say good morning to nursing staff
- Update your personal list of the firm's patients (new admissions, etc)
- Check patients' vitals, blood results and X-rays and have them handy
- Ask the nurses if anything happened overnight
- Have blank blood and X-ray forms handy for the ward round (unless the hospital ordering system is digitalised)

PRESENTING ON THE WARD ROUND

Presenting is an art form to try to perfect. Keep focused and present relevant positives and salient negatives only, but be prepared to answer any question asked (eg knowing who an elderly woman with a hip fracture lives with is important but need not be presented in the same breath as her current clinical status!). During a presentation, events should be given in a chronological sequence. The following is an example of how a patient should be presented:

[MR LG, FRACTURED LEFT ANKLE]

'This is Mr LG, a 28-year-old mechanic who was out drinking last night when, on leaving the pub, he stumbled and had a mechanical fall at approximately 1 am, resulting in an inversion injury to his left ankle. There was immediate swelling and pain with obvious deformity at the joint, and he was not able to weight-bear. He sustained no further injuries. He was brought to the A&E by ambulance. On examination, his vitals were all normal and his clinical status was stable. His ankle was deformed [describe] and there was bruising [state where]. The skin overlying the ankle was [breached/intact]. Pulses were [present/absent]. X-rays showed [describe; see Chapter 5a]. The fracture was manipulated under sedation and immobilised in a [type of plaster cast]. Besides his injury, he is a fit and healthy man with no other medical history and has been NBM since [time].'

Presentation time is about 5 minutes, giving plenty of time for questions!

OPERATING THEATRE: DOS AND DON'TS

DO have a good night's sleep and a proper breakfast before attending
DO review the relevant anatomy beforehand
DO ask the theatre sister to teach you how to scrub up properly (arrive early for this)
DO know the patients inside out *before* they arrive
DO make sure that there is a medical student scrubbed for *every* case
DO use time between cases wisely by either reviewing cases or practising knots
DON'T disturb the surgeon without asking permission first
DON'T annoy the scrub nurse: do as she says
DON'T chit-chat with other students during an operation if not scrubbed
DON'T touch instruments unless given explicit instruction to do so
DON'T look bored no matter how long and tedious the operation is

POST-OPERATIVE ROUND

If asked to present a patient on post-op rounds, don't panic. Start by stating the procedure the patient had and then use the following list of things that you should be interested in post-operatively:

- General clinical status of patient (alert, vomiting or in pain?)
- Examination (in particular, wound site, chest, calves and bowel sounds)
- Vital signs (look at trends as opposed to single values)
- Fluid charting and input-output balance (is the patient producing urine?)
- Drains (function and contents)
- Post-operative blood results
- Drug chart (receiving appropriate medications in the appropriate dosages?)

Have gloves for everyone handy in your pockets. Always be the first one to pick up the nursing chart and make a show of checking the vitals. Ask if wounds need to be observed and, if so, take the initiative to remove the dressing yourself (don't forget gloves!).

CHAPTER 3: GETTING STARTED: SURGICAL JARGON

SURGICAL ABBREVIATIONS

#	Fracture
1ry, 2ry, etc . . .	Primary, secondary, etc . . .
a/aa	artery/arteries
AA	Alcoholics Anonymous
ABG	Arterial blood gas
ABPI	Ankle-brachial pressure index
Ab/AdPL/B	Ab/ad-ductor pollicis longus/brevis
Abx	Antibiotics
AC	Air conduction
ACTH	Adrenocorticotrophic hormone
AF	Atrial fibrillation
AK[A]	Above knee [amputation]
AIDS	Acquired immunodeficiency syndrome
ALP	Alkaline phosphatase
Amp	Ampicillin
AOE	Acute otitis externa
AOM	Acute otitis media
AP	Antero–posterior X-ray
aPTT	Activated partial thromboplastin time
ARDS	Adult respiratory distress syndrome
ASA	Amino-salicylic acid (aspirin)
ASD	Atrial septal defect
ASIS	Anterior superior iliac spine
AST	Aspartate aminotransferase
AXR	Abdominal X-ray
BC	Bone conduction
bd	*bis die* (twice daily)
BE	Below elbow
BK[A]	Below knee [amputation]
BLS	Basic Life Support
BP	Blood pressure
CA	Carcinoma
CABG	Coronary artery bypass graft (cabbage)

CCF	Congestive cardiac failure
Cef	Cefuroxime
chrm	chromosome
CIS	Carcinoma in situ
CMV	Cytomegalovirus
C/O	Complains of
COPD	Chronic obstructive pulmonary disease
CRP	C-reactive protein (inflammatory marker)
CRT	Capillary refill time
CSOM	Chronic suppurative otitis media
CT	Computed tomography
CVA	Cerebrovascular accident (stroke is a better term)
CVP	Central venous pressure
CXR	Chest X-ray
D5W	Dextrose 5% in water
DHx	Drug history
DIC	Disseminated intravascular coagulation
DIPJ	Distal interphalangeal joint
DM	Diabetes mellitus
DRE	Digital rectal examination
DT	Delirium tremens
DVT	Deep vein thrombosis
Dx	Diagnosis
ECG	Electrocardiogram
Echo	Echocardiogram
ENT	Ear, nose & throat
EPB/L	Extensor pollicis brevis/longus
ESR	Erythrocyte sedimentation rate
ETOH	Alcohol
EUA	Examination under anaesthesia
Ex-Fix	External fixation
FBC	Full blood count
FDP	Fibrin degradation products
FDP/S	Flexor digitorum profundus/superficialis
FESS	Functional endoscopic sinus surgery
FFP	Fresh frozen plasma

FNA[C]	Fine needle aspirate [cytology]
FOOSH	Fall on the out-stretched hand
FTSG	Full thickness skin graft
GA	General anaesthetic
GCS	Glasgow Coma Scale
Gent	Gentamicin
GP	General Practitioner
G&S	Group & save
GTN	Glyceryl trinitrate
GXM	Group & cross match
HIV	Human immunodeficiency virus
HPV	Human papilloma virus
HTN	Hypertension
HZO	Herpes zoster ophthalmicus
ICP	Intracranial pressure
I&D	Incision & drainage (abscesses)
IHD	Ischaemic heart disease
IMN	Intramedullary nailing
IOP	Intra-ocular pressure
ITU	Intensive Therapy Unit
IVC	Inferior Vena Cava
IVDU	Intravenous drug user
IVF	Intravenous fluids
IVP/U	Intravenous pyelogram/urogram
JVP	Jugular venous pressure
KUB	Kidneys, ureters & bladder (plain film)
LA	Local anaesthetic
lat	Lateral X-ray
LFT	Liver function test
LUQ	Left upper quadrant
MAX FAX	Maxillo-facial surgery
MC	MetaCarpal
M/C/S	Microscopy, culture & sensitivity
Metro	Metronidazole
MI	Myocardial infarction
MOF	Multiorgan failure
MSU	Mid stream urine
MUA	Manipulation under anaesthetic

n/nn	Nerve/nerves
N/A	Not applicable
NAD	Nil abnormality detected
NBM	Nil By mouth
NGT	Nasogastric tube
NOF	Neck of femur
N/S	Normal saline
NSAIDs	Non-steroidal anti-inflammatory drugs
OA	Osteoarthritis
OCP	Oral contraceptive pill
od	*Omni die* (once daily)
qds	*Quater die sumendus* (4 times daily)
OGD	Oesophagastroduodenoscopy
OPG	OrthoPantoGram
ORIF	Open reduction and internal fixation
OT	Operating Theatre/Occupational Therapist
PAN	Polyarteritis nodosum
PCA	Patient controlled analgesia
PCWP	Pulmonary capillary wedge pressure
PDA	Patent ductus arteriosus
PE	Pulmonary embolism
PEEP	Positive end expiratory pressure
PERLA	Pupils equal and reactive to light and accommodation
PICU	Paediatric intensive therapy unit
PIPJ	Proximal interphalangeal joint
PMHx	Past medical history
PO	*Per os* (orally)
POP	Plaster of Paris
PR	*Per rectum* (rectally)
PRN	*Pro re nata* (as needed)
PSIS	Posterior superior iliac spine
PT	Prothrombin time
PTCA	Percutaneous transluminal coronary angioplasty
PUD	Peptic ulcer disease
PV	*Per vaginum* (vaginally)

qds	*Quater die sumendus* (to be taken 4 times daily)
qxh	Every *x* hours (eg q3h = every 3 hours)
RAPD	Relative afferent pupillary defect
RBS	Random blood sugar
r/o	Rule out
RTA	Road traffic accident
RUQ	Right upper quadrant
Rx	Treatment
SCC	Squamous cell carcinoma
SIRS	Systemic inflammatory response syndrome
SLE	Systemic lupus erythematosus
SNHL	SensoriNeural hearing loss
SOB	Shortness of breath
SSG	Split skin graft
stat	Immediately
STD	Sexually transmitted disease
SVC	Superior vena cava
Sx	Surgery
SXR	Skull X-ray
TB	Tuberculosis
tds	*Ter die sumendus* (to be taken 3 times daily)
TIA	Transient ischaemic attack
TM	Tympanic membrane
TMJ	TemporoMandibular joint
TOE	Transoesophegeal echocardiogram
TPN	Total parenteral nutrition
TRAM	Transverse rectus abdominis muscle
TTE	Trans-thoracic echocardiogram
UC	Ulcerative colitis
U&Es	Urea & electrolytes (and creatinine)
U/O	Urine output
URTI	Upper respiratory tract infection
USS	Ultrasound scan
UTI	Urinary tract infection

PART I

v/vv	Vein/veins
Vanc	Vancomycin
VE	Vaginal examination
VSD	Ventricular septal defect
VUJ	Vesico–ureteric junction
WBC/WCC	White blood cells/white cell count

GLOSSARY OF SURGICAL TERMINOLOGY

Abduct	Movement of any extremity *away* from the midline of the body
Adduct	Movement of any extremity *towards* the midline of the body
Adeno-	Pertaining to glands
Afferent	Toward
Anastomosis	Surgically created connection between two tubular structures (eg bowel, blood vessels, etc)
Angio-	Pertaining to blood vessels
Anomalous	Deviating from the norm
Aseptic	Complete absence of disease-causing micro-organisms.
Atelectasis	Alveolar collapse
Atresia	Congenital absence of abnormal narrowing of an opening or lumen (adj. **atretic**)
Biopsy	Tissue sample obtained and sent for histopathology
Cachexia	Generalised wasting associated with chronic disease or malignancy (adj. **cachectic**)
Calculus	Stone
Calor	One of the classic signs if inflammation; signifies warmth

Caseation	Breakdown of diseased tissue into cheese-like material (adj. **caseous**)
Caudal	Relating to lower part of the body
Chepal-	Pertaining to the head
Cicatrix	Scar
Colic	Pain which occurs in waves; usually occurs in tubular organs
Curettage	Scraping of the internal surface of an organ or body cavity with a spoon-line instrument (**curette**)
Cyst	Abnormal sac lined by epithelium and filled with fluid or semi-solid material
Diaphoresis	Excessive sweating
Diverticulum	A small sac or pouch projection from the wall of a hollow organ. The wall of a **true diverticulum** comprises all the layers of the parent organ (eg Meckel's diverticulum). The wall of a **pseudo-diverticulum** contains only some of the layers (eg diverticular disease of the colon)
Dolor	One of the classic signs of inflammation; signifies **pain**
Dysphagia	Difficulty swallowing (as opposed to **odynophagia** which is **painful** swallowing)
Ecchymosis	Bruising
-ectomy	Surgical removal (eg parotidectomy)
Epistaxis	Nosebleed
Excision biopsy	Biopsy in which entire tumour is removed
Fistula	An abnormal, **epithelialised** communication between two surfaces

Frequency	Abnormally increased urination
Functio laesa	One of the classic signs of inflammation; signifies **loss of function**
Haemangiona	Benign tumour of blood vessels
Haematemesis	Vomiting of blood
Haematoma	Blood clot within tissues which forms a solid mass. May resolve or become super-infected
Haematuria	Blood in the urine
Haemoptysis	Coughing-up of blood
Haemothorax	Blood within the pleural space
Hesitancy	Difficulty in initiating urination
Icterus	Jaundice
Incisional biopsy	Biopsy in which only a core of the tumour is removed
Induration	Abnormal hardening of a tissue or organ
Intussusception	Telescoping of one part of the bowel into adjacent bowel
Laparoscopy	Visualisation of peritoneal cavity with a laparoscope (makes use of fibre optics)
Laparotomy	Opening the abdominal cavity via a surgical incision
Lumen	Cavity within a tubular organ (adj. luminal)
Melaena	Black, tarry stool representing digested blood, most commonly occurring due to an upper GI bleed (must be more than 100 ml)
Nocturia	Abnormal urination at night usually interrupting sleep

Obstipation	Total failure to pass either flatus or stool
Odynophagia	Painful swallowing
Orchid-	Pertaining to the testicles
-orraphy	Surgical repair (eg herniorraphy)
-ostomy	Surgically created opening (eg colostomy) (from *stoma* which means mouth)
-otomy	Surgical incision into an organ (eg laparoscopy)
-pexy	Surgical fixation (eg orchidopexy)
Phlegmon	Solid, swollen, inflamed pancreatic tissue mass
Pneumaturia	Air in the urine (usually due to an **enterovesical fistula**)
Pneumothorax	Air within the pleural space
Pus	Fluid product of inflammation (see Chapter 25) (adj. **purulent**, not pussy!)
Rubor	One of the classic signs of inflammation; signifies **redness**
Sinus	Abnormal, blind-ending, epithelialised tract in an organ
Stenosis	Abnormal narrowing of a lumen, passage or opening
Suppuration	Formation of pus
Transection	Transverse division
Volar	Pertaining to surface of palm or sole

SURGICAL SIGNS, TESTS, LAWS, SYNDROMES AND EPONYMS

Allen's test

Test of hand circulation. Ask pt. to drain hand by forming a fist, and compress radial and ulnar aa. Ask pt. to open blanched fist. Release one artery and observe for palmar flushing (arterial patency). Repeat test for other artery

Argyll-Robinson's pupil

A pupil that contracts or expands to accommodate changes in focal length but does not respond to light. *Mnemonic:* **A**rgyll-**R**obinson **P**upil taken backwards then forward gives: **ARP, PRA**, which then translates to: **A**ccommodation **R**eflex **P**resent, **P**upillary **R**esponse **A**bsent

Barton's fracture

Fracture-dislocation of the distal radius, sometimes mistaken for a Colles' fracture. The fracture line runs across the volar lip of the radius and into the wrist joint. The hand and the fragment of distal radius undergo a proximal and volar displacement

Battle's sign

Periorbital ecchymoses in basal skull #

Beck's triad

Seen in cardiac tamponade. Consists of:
1. Jugular venous distension
2. Muffled heart sounds
3. ↓ BP

Bell's palsy

An acute lower motor neurone facial nerve palsy of unknown aetiology (diagnosis of exclusion)

Chvostek's sign

Seen in hypocalcaemia. Tapping over facial n. causes twitching of facial muscles

Colles' fracture

Fracture of the distal 2 cm of the radius with dorsal displacement of the distal fragment, giving characteristic **dinner-fork deformity**

Compartment syndrome

Condition of increased pressure in a confined anatomical space adversely affecting circulation and threatening the function and viability of tissues therein

Cushing's triad

Seen in raised ICP. Consists of:
1. ↑ BP
2. Bradycardia
3. Irregular respirations

DeQuervain's tenosynovitis

Inflammation of EPB and AbPL secondary to overuse. Elicited using **Finkelstein's test**

Finkelstein's test

Passive extension of the wrist with the thumb clenched in the fist, causing pain due to stretching of EPB and AbPL

Frey's syndrome

Warmth and sweating in the malar region of the face on eating or thinking or talking about food (syn. **gustatory sweating**). It may follow damage in the parotid region by trauma, mumps, purulent infection or parotidectomy. Following initial damage, autonomous fibres to salivary glands become re-connected in error with the sweat glands. Stimulus for salivation hence causes sweating and flushing. Flushing prevalent in females, sweating in males. **Gustatory tears** is also sometimes seen (syn. **crocodile tears**)

Galeazzi fracture

Radial shaft fracture with associated dislocation of the distal radioulnar joint, which disrupts the forearm axis joint (syn. **reverse Monteggia fracture**)

Gradenigo's syndrome

Seen in suppurative otitis media. Consists of:
1. Signs of acute suppurative otitis media
2. Ipsilateral abducens nerve palsy
3. Pain in the distribution of the ipsilateral trigeminal nerve

Histelberger's sign

Hyperaesthesia of the posterior external ear canal and ipsilateral hearing loss in acoustic neuroma

Horner's syndrome

Syndrome of the following ipsilateral signs:
1. Ptosis
2. Miosis (constricted pupil)
3. Anhidrosis (loss of sweating)
4. Enophthalmos
Caused by disruption of the ipsilateral sympathetic nerve supply to the eye (classically caused by **Pancoast tumour**, an upper lobe lung tumour)

Monteggia fracture

Dislocation of radial head with fracture of proximal 1/3 of the ulna

Osler–Rendu–Weber syndrome

Familial haemorrhagic telangiectasia causing telangiectasiae (spider naevi) in all mucosal surfaces, but most commonly presenting as epistaxis (still a rare cause!)

Pendred's syndrome

An autosomal recessive syndrome of congenital sensorineural hearing loss (SNHL) and a thyroid goitre

Pierre–Robin syndrome

Autosomal dominant condition consisting of the following:
1. Hypoplastic mandible
2. Cleft palate
3. Glossoptosis (downward displacement of the tongue which may cause obstructive sleep apnoea)
4. External, middle and inner ear problems

Raccoon eyes

Seen in basal skull #. Bilateral periorbital ecchymoses
(syn: **Panda eyes**)

Refsum's disease

A disease consisting of the following:
1. Retinitis pigmentosa
2. Cerebellar ataxia
3. Peripheral neuropathy
4. SNHL

Ramsay–Hunt syndrome

Facial nerve palsy caused by Herpes zoster infection of the facial nerve. Presents as a facial nerve palsy and painful, haemorrhagic blistering of the ipsilateral tympanic membrane (tympanica haemorrhagica)
(syn. **herpes zoster oticus**)

Smith's fracture

A fracture of the distal radius which occurs if the patient lands with the wrist in flexion. The radial fragment is displaced anteriorly, and the fracture does not extend into the joint
(syn. **reverse Colles' fracture**)

Superior vena cava syndrome

SVC obstruction (eg by tumour, thrombosis) causing engorged face, neck and upper chest veins (SVC distribution)

Thoracic outlet syndrome

Compression of structures exiting thoracic outlet (eg cervical rib)

PART I

Thornwald's cyst

A benign swelling of the nasopharynx, uncommon especially in adults. It is a cyst of the pharyngeal bursa located in the supero-posterior nasopharynx.
May cause occlusion of the orifice

Treacher–Collins syndrome

Hypoplasia of the maxilla and mandible with microtia (small ears) and external/inner ear problems (autosomal dominant)

Trousseau's sign

Seen in hypocalcaemia. Carpopedal spasm after blood occlusion (with BP cuff) in forearm or leg

Waardenburg's syndrome

An autosomal disorder consisting of the following:
1. Telecanthus [↑ distance between the inner corners of the eyes (the **canthi**; sing. canthus)]
2. Pigment disorder [**white forelock** and **heterochromia iridis** (different coloured irises)]
3. SNHL

PART II

Trauma & orthopaedics

CHAPTER 4: THE TRAUMA CALL IN ORTHOPAEDICS

What are the principles of ATLS?

Advanced **T**rauma **L**ife **S**upport principles advocate a thorough and reliable system of examination and initial resuscitation in order to identify and immediately treat potentially fatal injuries in trauma, followed by a more thorough and detailed assessment of the whole body leading eventually to complete and definitive care. These two processes are divided into a **primary** and **secondary** survey.

What is the primary survey?

It is the initial assessment of the trauma patient, designed to identify and treat life-threatening injuries immediately so that initial resuscitation is maximally effective. Remember assess **A,B,C,D and E**:
- **A**irway and cervical spine immobilisation
- **B**reathing (respiratory system)
- **C**irculation and haemorrhage control (**C**ardiovascular system)
- **D**isability
- **E**xposure

What life-threatening injuries *must* be identified and treated in the primary survey?

Mnemonic: **ATOMIC**
Airway compromise resulting in inadequate ventilation
Tension pneumothorax
Open pneumothorax/sucking chest wound
Massive haemothorax
Incipient flail chest
Cardiac tamponade

What are the aims of the secondary survey?	A thorough head to toe assessment after initial resuscitation to identify all injuries caused by trauma and outline a plan for full treatment and definitive care
What X-rays are included in a standard trauma series?	The following films: 1. C-spine 2. CXR 3. Pelvic XR

THE PRIMARY SURVEY

AIRWAY AND C-SPINE CONTROL

Who is at risk of C-spine injury and subsequent neurological damage?	All patients involved in trauma must be assumed to have an unstable C-spine # until excluded clinically and radiologically
How is the C-spine initially managed?	In the following ways: 1. **C-spine hard collar**: reduces voluntary movement by around 30% 2. **Bilateral sandbags/struts** taped across bed to secure hard collar in fixed position Suboptimal immobilisation in a hard collar only is used in a restless agitated patient, as this is preferred to splinting the C-spine of a thrashing torso/lower body
How is the C-spine definitively investigated?	With radiological assessment which includes the following three views: 1. Lateral C-spine: picks up 80% of C-spine injuries. Must include all seven cervical vertebrae *and* the C7–T1 junction to be an **adequate film** 2. AP view – picks up 95% of bony injuries when combined with the lateral view

3. Open mouth/odontoid peg view – picks up 99% of injuries when used with above views

Further management is based on findings and includes flexion-extension views and CT scanning.

What types of injuries compromise the airway?

Two main groups:

1. **Facial/neck trauma**: stab wounds to the neck, facial trauma post-assault or unrestrained passengers in head-on collisions, causing oropharyngeal loose bodies/haematoma/bruising

2. **Head injury with low GCS and impaired laryngeal/pharyngeal reflexes**: GCS < 8 with impaired cough or gag reflex implies inability to self protect the airway against aspiration of vomit/blood. The airway must therefore be cleared and secured

How is the airway evaluated?

Ask a simple question. A lucid response in a normal voice implies an intact airway with no laryngeal compromise. If no response:

Look: for any misting of the oxygen mask, facial trauma, blood or foreign bodies in the oropharynx and signs of any ventilatory obstruction, such as tracheal tug, see-saw breathing (abdominal retraction on inspiration with no chest movement) or complete apnoea/cyanosis

Listen: for signs of air movement, cough reflex and evidence of upper airway obstruction such as:

• Stridor (hoarse inspiratory sound caused by extrathoracic large airway obstruction)
• Gurgling

PART II

- Wheeze (expiratory sound caused by intrathoracic small airway obstruction – implies pathology within chest rather than at airway level)

Feel: for breath on your cheek; assess chest expansion/symmetry at the same time by looking down the chest wall. Gag reflex can also be tested with utilisation of airway adjuncts (see below)

What basic airway manoeuvres do you know of?

1. Head tilt, chin lift: suitable only when there is *no suspicion* of C-spine injury
2. Jaw thrust
3. Yankauer suction of blood/liquid obstructing airway

If these fail, what next?

Use an airway adjunct

What types do you know of?

1. McGill forceps: angled forceps used to retrieve obstructing foreign bodies
2. Nasopharyngeal airway: contraindicated with suspicion of basal skull or cribriform plate #s; or severe nasal trauma (risk of creating **false passage**)
3. Oropharyngeal (Guedel) airway

How would you definitively secure the airway?

Endotracheal (ET) tube placement

BREATHING

When should the team assess breathing?

Only when the airway has been cleared and secured

What type of injuries compromise breathing?

Three categories:
1. **Blunt trauma**:
   - Direct impact
   - Shear forces (if a patient is run over by a motor vehicle)

- Deceleration injuries (high-speed RTA/fall from height)

2. **Penetrating trauma**:
   - Stab wounds
   - Gun shot wounds (GSW)
3. **Blast injuries**: a proximal explosion results in pulmonary damage secondary to capillary haemorrhage and alveolar rupture

How is breathing assessed?

Look:
- Cyanosis
- Increased respiratory rate
- Asymmetrical chest expansion
- Use of accessory muscles/tracheal tug/increased work of breathing
- Paradoxical chest wall movement (a section of the chest wall moving inwards on inspiration, secondary to multiple rib fractures)
- Superficial signs of trauma (bruising, GSW, stab wounds, seatbelt marks)

Listen:
- Areas of inadequate air entry (all zones must be auscultated)
- Bronchial breathing
- Wheeze (bronchospasm secondary to intrathoracic injury)

Feel:
- Air movement (is the patient breathing spontaneously?)
- Tracheal deviation
- Percuss chest for dullness/hyperresonant areas
- Subcutaneous emphysema (a sign of likely pneumothorax with parietal pleura rupture)

What life-threatening problems must be excluded immediately?

The following:

1. **Tension pneumothorax**: build up of air under pressure in the thoracic cavity, compressing the ipsilateral lung and displacing the mediastinal contents and contralateral lung.
   Occurs due to a one-way valve mechanism introducing air on inspiration, but blocking its release during expiration

2. **Open pneumothorax**: open chest wall wound connected to the thoracic cavity. If chest wall deficit is of a significant diameter, air will follow the path of least resistance and enter the thoracic cavity here on inspiration, rather than down the trachea. Syn. **sucking chest wound** due to the noise produced as the above occurs

3. **Massive haemothorax**: collection of >1500 ml blood in the thoracic cavity secondary to intercostal artery/large vessel rupture

4. **Flail chest**: multiple rib fractures causing a portion of the chest wall to **move paradoxically inwards** on inspiration due to a lack of continuity with the remaining bony chest wall

How are these conditions detected clinically?

Must have a high index of suspicion. Also, obvious distress and hypoxia, and the following during the primary survey:

Tension pneumothorax:
- Decreased ipsilateral chest expansion

- Tracheal deviation to contralateral side
- Hyperresonance to percussion over ipsilateral side
- Decreased ipsilateral air entry on auscultation
- Tachycardia, tachypnoea and distended neck veins

Open pneumothorax:
- Obvious chest wall defect with sucking noise on inspiration
- Decreased air entry and expansion on ipsilateral side
- Tachycardia and tachypnoea

Massive haemothorax:
- Decreased ipsilateral chest expansion
- Dull percussion note on the ipsilateral side
- Decreased air entry on the ipsilateral side
- Tachypnoea, tachycardia and signs of hypovolaemia

Flail chest:
- Paradoxical chest wall movement
- Crepitus on palpation of damaged area
- Decreased air entry on ipsilateral side
- Tachypnoea and tachycardia

PART II

How is tension pneumothorax treated?

Immediately by decompression by needle thoracocentesis, then definitively by chest drain insertion (thoracostomy) at a later stage

What are the anatomical landmarks for thoracocentesis?

2nd intercostal space at the manubriosternal junction in the mid-clavicular line

What are the anatomical landmarks for chest drain insertion?

5th intercostal space, mid-axial line

How is open pneumothorax treated?

Occlusive dressing is applied to the sucking wound and taped on **three sides only**. This creates a one-way valve, through which expired air can escape, but limits air entry to the thoracic cavity.

Followed by chest drain insertion on the ipsilateral side at a clean site away from wound.

What further investigations should be obtained?

Blood investigations:
1. GXM: for transfusion as necessary
2. ABG: provides invaluable information regarding oxygenation and lung function as well as an **immediate Hb estimation**. Can also provide **carboxyhaemoglobin** estimation in cases of smoke inhalation

Imaging:

CXR: still the most important:

Pneumothorax: loss of outer lung markings (1 cm rim of lucency approx. equal to 10% loss of lung volume)

Haemothorax: blunting of costophrenic angle on erect chest implies 300–400 ml blood in the pleural space

Also in diagnosis of contusion, parenchymal injury and other pathology

CT scan: used as necessary to provide specific information only in a patient stable for transfer and after the secondary survey

CIRCULATION

What is shock?

Shock is the clinically used term for a **compromise in circulation** leading to **inadequate tissue perfusion**. Metabolic demands of the body are not met leading to abnormal physiology

What types of shock are there?

There are five types:
1. **Hypovolaemic**: low intravascular volume, eg in haemorrhage
2. **Cardiogenic**: failure of the heart as a pumping mechanism due to 1ry damage and/or 2ry cardiac tamponade
3. **Septic**: maldistribution of fluid due to the action of chemical messengers during the inflammatory process of infection
4. **Neurogenic**: maldistribution of fluid due to loss of muscle tone/ nerve signals; eg in transection of the spinal cord
5. **Anaphylactic**: maldistribution of fluid due to allergic stimulus and cytokine release

What do they all have in common?

Intravascular fluid volume is no longer adequate to transport oxygen to the tissues for cellular uptake and aerobic metabolism

In a shocked patient, which type is assumed until proven otherwise?

Hypovolaemic 2ry to haemorrhage

What types of haemorrhage do you know?

There are two types:
1. **Obvious haemorrhage**:
   - Compound fractures
   - Digital/limb amputation
   - Arterial puncture wounds

2. **'Hidden' haemorrhage**:
   - Long bone fractures (closed)
   - Thoracic trauma (collects in thoracic cavity)
   - Abdominal trauma (intra/extra peritoneal)
   - Pelvic fractures (closed)

Which wounds must be treated with a high index of suspicion?

Penetrating wounds to the neck and mediastinum (risk of large vessel puncture or cardiac puncture leading to tamponade or cardiogenic shock)

How is shock clinically assessed?

Look:
- Peripheral/central cyanosis ($\downarrow$ perfusion)
- Patient cold and clammy (**'shut down'** due to peripheral vasoconstriction as a sympathetic response to haemorrhage)
- Distended jugular veins (cardiogenic shock)
- Visible trauma with/without haemorrhage
- Respiratory rate (normally 14–20 breaths/min in adult)
- Evidence of confusion, aggression, drowsiness or coma (cerebral hypoxia)
- Jugular venous pulse (JVP) wave if present (this is a tricky sign in any situation and so its use in the rapid assessment of a trauma patient is minimal)

Listen:
- Muffled heart sounds over the appropriate areas

Feel:
- Pulse: note **rate** (normal 60–100 bpm), **rhythm** (regular/irregular) and **volume** (bounding, thready, absent). If radial pulse absent, try carotid and femoral arteries. No pulse indicates **cardiac arrest** and BLS should be commenced
- Capillary refill time (CRT): press on sternum for 5 s. The area should blanch and return to normal colour in less than 2 s. Longer implies shock

What *must* also be performed?

The following bedside investigations:
- Blood pressure
- Oxygen saturations
- Cardiac monitoring and rhythm trace
- Urine output (usually as part of the secondary survey post catheterisation)

How can this information be used to assess blood loss in a patient in haemorrhagic shock?

See Table 4.1. It is based on the average 70-kg man with a 5 l intravascular volume

PART II

Table 4.1

	Class 1	Class 2	Class 3	Class 4
BP Systolic Diastolic	Unchanged Unchanged	Normal Raised	Reduced Reduced	Very low Very low/ unrecordable
Pulse bpm Volume	High normal Normal	100–120 Normal	>120 Thready	>120 Very thready
CRT	Normal	Slow (>2 s)	Slow (>2 s)	Undetectable
Respiratory rate	Normal	Tachypnoea	>20/min	>20/min
Urine output	>30 ml/h	20–30 ml/h	10–20 ml/h	0–10 ml/h
Extremities	Normal colour	Pale	Pale	Pale, clammy
Complexion	Normal	Pale	Pale	Ashen
Mental state	Alert	Anxious	Aggressive/ drowsy	Drowsy/ confused
Blood loss (like game of tennis) % Volume	Love-fifteen <15% 750 ml	Fifteen-thirty 15–30% 800–1500 ml	Thirty-forty 30–40% 1500–2000 ml	Game over! >40% >2000 ml

How is shock managed?

As hypovolaemic shock until proven otherwise: with rapid intravascular volume repletion (fluids)

So how would you treat this?

In the following steps:

1. Intravenous access via two wide-bore cannulae (14G ideally) in the antecubital fossa
2. *Failing this*: cannulation of any forearm veins with the widest bore possible
3. *Failing this*: a surgical 'cut down' (direct exposure of a accessible vein via dissection); saphenous vein most commonly used

4. *In kids, if 1 & 2* fail: intraosseous access can be attempted at the tibial tuberosity (*not* adults!)

NB Immediate central venous access with a large-bore cannula or via the Seldinger technique may be used first in experienced hands. Otherwise, it is used when peripheral access is impossible

Initial replacement should then be commenced with a 10- to 20-ml/kg bolus of warmed fluid via a pressure bag

What is your 1st choice of fluid?

Hartman's solution

What is the Seldinger technique?

A needle is inserted into central vein (jugular or subclavian), and a guidewire threaded through it. Needle is removed, and a cannula is threaded over the wire into the vein and secured

What should be done after cannulation but *before* starting fluids?

Collect 20 ml blood for:
1. G&S (or GXM depending on clinical scenario)
2. FBC: baseline
3. U&Es: baseline
4. Glucose estimation (via BM machine preferentially or lab glucose)
4. Serum save (for future tests as needed, forensic or otherwise)

PART II

What else must also be done?

The following adjunctive measures:

1. Adequate oxygenation (hence why B comes before C in the ABCDEs!). No benefit in restoring circulation if hypoxia continues, due to inadequate ventilation/oxygenation of blood at lungs: give as much O_2 therapy as possible, via intubation if necessary

2. Control of external haemorrhage:
   - Direct pressure onto bleeding area
   - Elevation of injured limb
   - Head-down tilt to maximise cerebral perfusion

What types of fluids are used in shock?

The following are available:

1. Hartman's solution (syn. **Ringer's lactate**)
2. Other crystalloids (eg normal saline)
3. Colloids (gelatin solutions): high osmotic load thought to give greater intravascular volume expansion
4. Blood products: provide oxygen transport, unlike any of above fluids

When is blood indicated?

In ongoing fluid loss and with class 3–4 shock (30–40% blood loss)

What type of blood should be used?

Depends on the clinical scenario and condition of the patient on arrival:

Needed immediately: *O -ve (universal donor)*

- Packed rhesus negative (Rh -ve) type-O red cells with no surface AB antigen and no anti A or anti B plasma

- Not cross-matched, therefore mild/moderate transfusion reactions unrelated to ABO rhesus system may occur

Needed quickly (5–10 min): *Type specific*

- ABO typed to match recipient's blood type
- Not fully cross-matched for other antigens
- Requires serum sample of pt's blood to the lab

Needed within 30–60 min: *Fully cross-matched*

- ABO and antibody screened to ensure maximum compatibility with recipient
- Requires serum sample of pt's blood to the lab

Once initial shock treatment has begun, what next?	Directed treatment of the actual cause of shock
What life-threatening circulatory condition must be identified and treated during the 1ry survey?	**Cardiac tamponade**: accumulation of blood within the fibrous pericardial sac (usually 2ry to myocardial trauma). This exerts external pressure on the heart and interferes with diastolic filling and subsequent ventricular ejection
How is cardiac tamponade recognised?	**Beck's triad**: 1. Hypotension 2. Muffled heart sounds 3. Raised JVP Also, **Kussmaul's sign**: raised JVP on inspiration due to impeded venous return
What is cardiac tamponade a diagnosis of?	Exclusion. Usually diagnosed when inserting bilateral chest drains for a haemothorax results in no clinical improvement

PART II

What is the management of cardiac tamponade?

ABCs (*always say this first!*), followed by 1 of 2 options:
1. Emergency pericardiocentesis (aspiration of blood from pericardial sac)
2. Emergency room thoracotomy (open evacuation of pericardial sac $\pm$ 1ry repair of wound)

When should a ER thoracotomy be done?

In the following circumstances:
1. Penetrating trauma to the chest (especially pericardiac) with established vital signs initially, followed by marked clinical deterioration
2. Uncontrollable life-threatening intra hilar haemorrhage, requiring cross-clamping as an emergency measure prior to theatre

What are the contraindications?

Numerous, but include:
- Blunt trauma
- >10 min CPR
- All patients with no established vital signs at the scene

DISABILITY

How would you immediately assess neurological status?

The **AVPU** system in the immediate, followed by the definitive Glasgow Coma Scale (**GCS**):

AVPU:

A: Spontaneously **A**lert (equivalent to GCS 14–15)

V: Responsive to **V**oice (equivalent to GCS 9–10)

P: Responsive to **P**ain (equivalent to GCS 7–8)

U: **U**nresponsive (equivalent to GCS of 3)

GCS: comprises three elements and scored by best possible response to give a total out of 15:

Best eye response
- No response [1]
- Eye opening to painful stimuli [2]
- Eye opening to verbal stimuli [3]
- Spontaneous eye opening [4]

Best verbal response
- No verbal response [1]
- Incomprehensible (noises) [2]
- Inappropriate (words only) [3]
- Confused (talking in sentences) [4]
- Orientated and lucid response [5]

Best motor response
- No response [1]
- Decerebrate [2]
- Decorticate [3]
- Withdrawal to pain [4]
- Localising to pain [5]
- Following commands [6]

PART II

What is the highest GCS score?

15: pt. fully alert, awake and aware

What is the lowest GCS score?

3 (*not zero!*): pt. comatose/ unresponsive

At what GCS score should a patient be intubated?

8

How often should the GCS be repeated in trauma?

Every 15 min. Document every time!

EXPOSURE

How much of the patient should be exposed?

All! The patient should be fully exposed from head to toe to note any injuries at any points on the body (use shears if necessary)

Why?

Visual clues may exist after full exposure, eg seatbelt marks indicating possible sternal trauma

What *must* be done on exposure?

A log-roll (pt. rolled onto side whilst maintaining spinal immobility; requires up to 5 people)

What is assessed on log-roll?

Back, buttocks, thighs and posterior legs and spine (deformities, focal tenderness, ecchymoses).
A DRE *must* be done.

What information is gained on DRE?

1. Anal tone ($\downarrow$ in cord trauma)
2. Blood (anorectal/pelvic trauma)
3. Prostate (high-riding prostate suggests urethral rupture)
4. Bony spicules (pelvic fracture)

What must be avoided in the exposed patient?

Hypothermia. Insulation is a *must* following log-roll

How is core body temperature most accurately assessed?

Rectally

How can core temperature be raised in hypothermia?

1. Bair Huggers® and covering (mild hypothermia)
2. Warmed fluid instituted into bodily orifices:
   - IV fluids
   - Orogastric
   - Intravesical
   - Intraperitoneal
   - Rectal

SECONDARY SURVEY

What are the essential objectives of the secondary survey?

Having addressed and treated any immediate life-threatening injuries, the secondary survey refers to a definitive history, thorough examination and formation of a management plan:
- Examination from head to toe, front and back
- 'Fingers and tubes in every orifice'
- Incident and collateral history

- Complete medical history
- Assimilation of all directed investigations
- Formulation of a definitive management plan

What investigations should be done in the secondary survey?

Any relevant ones. At the very least a trauma series should be obtained, together with basic blood tests and an ECG

What history should you take?

1. Paramedic handover
2. Collateral witness history
3. Patient's history
4. **AMPLE** medical history
   Allergies
   Medications
   Past medical history
   Last meal
   Events leading to situation

What happens if a change of deterioration in a patient's clinical condition occurs?

Return to assessment of ABCDE immediately and evaluate/treat as necessary until the patient's stability allows them to proceed with the secondary survey

PELVIS

What specific findings on clinical examination may imply pelvic injury?

The following:
1. Obvious deformity or compound injury
2. Localised pain/limb paraesthesia
3. Signs of retroperitoneal haemorrhage: bruising of scrotum, buttocks or along the line of inguinal ligament (**Fox's sign**)
4. Signs of urethral injury: blood at urethral meatus, high riding prostate, inability to void

PART II

5. Rectal examination: blood and palpable bony fragments; decreased anal tone implying neurological and lumbosacral injury
6. Abnormal assessment of stability

What different types of pelvic injury do you know of?

Three major patterns of injury exist, depending on the direction of force exerted on the hemipelvis:

1. **External rotation of the hemipelvis with disruption of the pubic symphysis (AP compression)**; caused by one of the following:
   a. Caused by direct AP compression force
   b. Caused by direct posterior blow to the iliac spines
   c. Caused by forced external rotation of the lower limb
2. **Internal rotation of the hemipelvis with compression fractures at the pubic rami (lateral compression)**; caused by lateral impact and medial compression
3. **Vertical shear with fracture dislocation of the hemipelvis and superoposterior displacement**; caused by vertical load fracturing pubic rami and sacroiliac joint with displacement as above

What is pelvic springing?

A basic clinical test to assess stability and integrity of the pelvic ring:
- Involves gentle compression of the iliac wings
- Designed to reveal pelvic instability to clinically suggest a fracture prior to imaging

What is the main concern in pelvic fracture?

Uncontrolled haemorrhage into the pelvic cavity, which can store litres

What interim measures are available for unstable pelvic fractures in the resus room?

1. Using a sheet placed under the buttocks, the ends can be brought anteriorly and knotted to provide a basic splint
2. External surgical fixation:
   - **Anterior external fixation** involves 2 pin insertions into the anterior border of the ilium bilaterally, with rigid interconnecting frame
   - **Posterior external fixation** involves pin insertion in the line between ASIS and PSIS and connection of these pins via reducing clamp

Should be carried out by an experienced orthopaedic surgeon due to risks of iatrogenic neurovascular damage

MUSCULOSKELETAL

What musculoskeletal injuries can contribute to shock?

1. Arterial bleed
2. Pelvic fracture
3. Large vessel puncture
4. Limb amputation
5. Long bone fracture
   a. Humerus: blood loss 0.5–1.5 l
   b. Tibia: blood loss 0.5–1.5 l
   c. Femur: blood loss 1.0–2.5 l

How should the musculoskeletal system be approached in the secondary survey?

As always, **ABCs first!!** Once patient is stable, the following can be taken into account:

History:
- Position of patient on their arrival
- Obvious/suspected trauma
- Seatbelt/airbag/mobilisation after RTA
- Direction of impact
- Found near/away from the site of the accident
- Remember to take an 'AMPLE' history; also important: previous joint/limb pathology and osteoporosis/osteopenia (increases susceptibility to trauma)

Look: expose patient fully and compare both sides for:
- Open fractures (exposed bone – may not be immediately obvious)
- Swelling
- Deformity
- Bruising
- Wounds
- Colour of limbs distal to injury

Feel: compare both sides for:
- Temperature of the distal limb
- Crepitus
- Joint effusions/haemarthroses
- Capillary refill time
- Pain in the conscious patient
- Neurological integrity – fine touch/motor function and hidrosis (skin sweating)

Move: compare both sides for:
- Range of active movement in the conscious patient
- Passive movement in the unconscious patient; *an obvious or suspected # should not be manipulated until X-ray, as this will in no way add to diagnosis – joint dislocations should be reduced as soon as possible though*
- Weight bearing as tolerated if applicable

What investigations should be ordered?

Standard X-rays for simple trauma (see next question)

What is the 'rule of twos'?

When ordering an X-ray:
1. Consider **2 joints**: the joints above and below any identified injury
2. **2 views** (AP and lateral) of each fracture to accurately note displacement and angulation
3. If any doubt remains, X-ray **2 sides** (injured side and contralateral side for comparison; rarely done)

PART II

CHAPTER 5: FRACTURES

GENERAL APPROACH

What types of joints do you know of?

Hip joint: a **ball-and-socket**:
- Formed by acetabulum (pelvis) and femoral head
- Covered by synovium
- Capsule (main blood supply)
- Ligaments (stability)
- Muscles (movement)
- Movements (flexion/extension, abduction/adduction, internal/external rotation)

Knee joint: a **hinge joint** where movements are flexion and extension:
- Formed by the lower end of the femur and the upper end of the tibia and the patella anteriorly
- Covered by synovium
- Capsule (blood supply)
- Quadriceps attach to the patella (extension)
- Patella ligament attached to the top of the tibia (extension)
- Hamstring muscles (flexion)
- Neurovascular structures posteriorly
- Medial and lateral collateral ligaments (stability)
- Medial and lateral menisci (act as shock absorbers)
- Anterior and posterior cruciate ligaments (stability)

Ankle joint: also a **hinge joint** formed by lower tibia and fibula and upper end of the talus:
- Covered by synovium
- Capsule (blood supply)

- Anterior muscles for dorsiflexion (including tib. ant. and ext. digitorum)
- Posterior muscles for plantarflexion (gastrocnemius/soleus complex)
- Medial muscles for inversion (including tibialis posterior)
- Lateral muscles for eversion (including peroneii)
- Ligaments (medial and lateral)
- Movements (dorsiflexion/plantarflexion)

Subtalar joint: formed by talus above and calcaneum (heel bone) below:

- Rich blood supply
- Number of ligaments
- Movements (inversion/eversion)

How are #s caused?

By the following mechanisms (amongst others):

1. Falls (low energy trauma)
2. RTA (high energy trauma)
3. Sports injuries
4. Stress fractures
5. Pathological conditions (bone cancer/metastases)

What are open and closed #s?

Closed: the bone has #d without breaching the skin (syn. **simple #**)

Open: the bone has #d and breached the skin making it susceptible to infection (syn. **compound #**). Open fractures are an emergency. The wound should be photographed and then immediately irrigated with saline in A&E. It should then be covered with Betadine-soaked gauzes and the limb splinted. Intravenous antibiotics should be commenced immediately and tetanus status should be checked and appropriate prophylaxis given. Radiographs are made of the injury and the patient must be taken as soon as possible to the operating theatre for debridement, irrigation and fracture stabilisation. The wound is subsequently re-inspected every 2–3 days until it can be definitively closed.

How are #s managed?

Either **non-operatively** or **operatively**

Non-operative: A simple non-displaced fracture needs either a splint or a plaster for a short period of time (eg green stick fracture in a child)

Fractures with displacement require manipulation under local, regional or general anaesthetic. The reduced fracture needs to be held in a plaster until the fracture heals

Operative: may require **internal** or **external fixation**. The indications are:

1. Failed conservative treatment
2. Polytrauma patients
3. Fractures with neurovascular trauma
4. Fractures involving the joint (articular fractures)
5. Pathological fractures (eg osteoporotic hip fractures in the elderly)
6. Some complex fractures (eg fractures of the femur, talus and forearm)

Can you give some examples of internal fixation?

1. Plate and screws
2. Intramedullary nail
3. Kirschner wires (K-wires)

PART II

When is external fixation used?

In open (compound) #s. An Ex-Fix is used to reduce the fracture externally, hence avoiding open surgery and keeping away from the open wound, in the hope of reducing infection risk to the fracture site

What complications of #s?

There are many! Group them as follows to help yourself to remember:

General:
1. Haemorrhage and shock
2. Thromboembolism
3. Fat embolism
4. Chest complications (eg chest infection)
5. Urinary complications (eg urinary tract infection)
6. Pressure sores

Specific:

Related to fracture
1. Delayed union of fracture
2. Malunion (deformity)
3. Infection (especially with open #s)
4. Joint stiffness (prolonged immobilisation and #s involving joints)
5. Compartment syndrome (tibia #, supracondylar #s in children)
6. Neurovascular complications
7. Avascular necrosis (especially with femoral head, humeral head, talus, scaphoid)

Related to treatment
1. Damage to soft tissue (eg skin)
2. Damage to neurovascular structures
3. Damage to tendons and muscles
4. Breakage of screws and rods
5. Pin track infection (especially with Ex-Fix)
6. Further surgical procedure to remove metal

UPPER LIMB INJURIES

What is the most common injury associated with upper limb #s?

Fall on the out-stretched hand (FOOSH)

What main #s are associated with FOOSH?

Start distally and move proximally: you'll remember most of them this way!

Wrist (carpal aspect):
1. Scaphoid #
2. Lunate dislocation
3. Perilunate dislocation

Wrist (radio-ulnar aspect):
1. Colles'/Colles'-type #

Forearm:
1. Mid-shaft radio-ulnar #
2. Monteggia #
3. Galeazzi #

Elbow:
1. Radial head #/dislocation
2. Supracondylar #
3. Elbow dislocation

Humerus:
1. Mid-shaft humeral #

Shoulder:
1. Anterior shoulder dislocation
2. Surgical neck of humerus #
3. Clavicular #
4. Sternoclavicular dislocation

SCAPHOID FRACTURE

Which is the most commonly #d carpal bone?

The scaphoid

What parts is the scaphoid bone divided up into?

Proximal and distal segments separated by its waist

Where does it usually #?

Through its **waist**

What is its claim to fame?

One of the bones in the body which may undergo **avascular necrosis (AVN)** following fracture

Which other ones may undergo AVN following #?	The **talus** in the foot, the **femoral head** and the **humeral head**
What makes the scaphoid bone prone to AVN?	Its blood supply is an end artery which runs from distal to proximal
Which anatomical part is most prone to AVN?	The **proximal pole**
Why?	The blood supply enters the *distal* pole, supplying this end and travelling proximally towards the proximal pole. Fracture through the waist compromises the blood supply of the *proximal* pole
What will AVN lead to?	Eventual osteoarthritis at the carpo-radial joint
Profile?	***History****:* FOOSH ***Examination****:* tenderness in the **anatomical snuffbox** (region bounded by the tendons of the abductor pollicis longus and extensor pollicis brevis laterally, and the extensor pollicis longus medially; contains the scaphoid bone and radial artery), and pain on **telescoping** the thumb (**Chen's scaphoid compression test** – force applied axially along the thumb; pain caused by metacarpal of thumb hitting the injured scaphoid bone with which it articulates) ***Radiology****:* ask for **scaphoid views**; # may be obvious, but often isn't. Re-X-ray in 2/52 when # becomes more obvious due to osteopenia around the # ***Treatment****:* treat symptomatically if # not obvious on initials film; scaphoid plaster for at least 6/52 with hand held in the **cup-holding** position for confirmed #

LUNATE AND PERILUNATE DISLOCATION

Of these, which one is considered an orthopaedic emergency?

Lunate dislocation: lunate dislocates in a volar direction and can exert pressure on the median nerve leading to median nerve palsy

How does it present?

History: FOOSH
Examination: swelling/ecchymosis at wrist ± median nerve symptoms (including paraesthesia of radial 3 1/2 fingers and weakness of AbPB)
Radiology: on **lat,** lunate should look like a **cup** holding the rest of the carpus within it like an **apple** (**apple in a cup** sign); this is lost as lunate cup has flipped in a volar direction
Treatment: attempt immediate reduction under analgesia/sedation ± ORIF. Immobilise in plaster for 6/52

What about perilunate dislocation?

Very unstable injury, but much less risk of median n. injury than lunate dislocation

How does it present?

History: FOOSH
Examination: obvious deformity at wrist with swelling ± ecchymoses. May have paraesthesia in distribution of median nerve if dislocation has caused n. to become stretched
Radiology: obvious dislocation of carpus with lunate in its normal position; on lat, apple is out of cup, but cup remains upright
Treatment: reduction under sedation + BE slab; may need K-wires ± ORIF. Treat in plaster for 6/52

How are the carpal bones remembered?	*Mnemonic:* **Some Lovers Try Positions That They Can't Handle** (from radial to ulnar, proximal row of bones first): **S**caphoid **L**unate **T**riquetrum **P**isiform **T**rapezium **T**rapezoid **C**apitate **H**amate

COLLES'/COLLES'-TYPE FRACTURE

What is the definition of a Colles' #?	A # of the distal 1 inch of the radius *occurring in osteoporotic bone* with displacement and/or angulation of the distal fragment dorsally and radially. There may also be **impaction** of the fracture fragments, **shortening**, and an **associated fracture of the ulna styloid**
What is a Colles'-type # then?	Exactly the same type of # as a Colles' #, but occurring in non-osteoporotic bone
How do they present?	*History:* FOOSH *Examination:* a deformed distal radius, classically giving a **dinner-fork deformity** due to its resemblance to one. May be swelling/ecchymosis. *Radiology:* # of distal end of radius with displacement and/or angulation of the distal fragment dorsally and radially. Look for another associated fracture (see above) *Treatment:* reduction (under haematoma block or sedation) of distal fragment using a combination of longitudinal traction, ulnar

deviation, wrist flexion and counter-traction at the elbow. Place in a BE slab in wrist flexion and ulnar deviation. K-wiring ± ORIF may become necessary if closed reduction unsatisfactory. Treat in plaster for 5–6/52

MID-SHAFT RADIO-ULNAR FRACTURE

What types of forearm #s may occur during FOOSH?

Isolated radial or ulnar #s or a combined radio-ulnar #

How do they present?

History: usually FOOSH
Examination: deformed forearm with swelling ± ecchymosis; look out for compound #! If only 1 of the bones is #d, overall deformity may be slight as other intact bone struts the forearm in a relatively normal position
Radiology: obvious # of forearm bone(s)
Management: depends on severity of #.
Generally:
Closed #/no displacement: AE plaster
Closed #/minimally displaced: MUA and AE plaster
Closed #/grossly displaced: ORIF (plating or flexible intramedullary nailing in children)
Open #: Ex-Fix

What are the risks of mid-shaft radio-ulnar #s?

The following can occur if both bones are #d:

1. **Compartment syndrome** due to gross swelling which can occur (see 'Compartment syndrome', below)

PART II

57

2. **Malunion**, esp. with closed reduction, causing future problems with pronation/supination
3. **Delayed/non-union**, which will require bone grafting/plating (see 'General approach' above)

If only 1 bone is #d, look out for **non-union**, as the other intact bone can strut the ends of the #d bone apart

What would you do if there was an open #?

Ex-Fix (see 'General approach' above)

MONTEGGIA AND GALEAZZI FRACTURES

What is a Monteggia #?

It is a combination of the following 2 injuries centred around the **proximal forearm** region:
1. # of upper ⅓ of **ulna** with angulation and shortening
2. **Radial head** dislocation (most commonly anterior, ie in a volar direction)

What is a Galeazzi #?

It is a combination of the following 2 injuries centred around the **distal forearm** region:
1. # of lower ⅓ of **radius**
2. **Distal radio-ulnar joint** dislocation (ulnar head juts out at dorsal aspect of wrist)

How do they present?

History: **Monteggia**: direct blow to forearm (more common) or FOOSH; **Galeazzi**: FOOSH, usually with elbow flexed

Examination: difficult to diagnose clinically; deformity and swelling present

Radiology: specific injuries will be seen; a **true lat** will be necessary to see radial head dislocation in Monteggia #

Treatment: ORIF in both types: involves the 2 following steps:

1. Plating the #, hence restoring original bone length
2. Reducing the dislocation (which usually occurs spontaneously after restoring bone length)

How can the differences between the 2 #s be remembered?

Mnemonic: **MURG**
This mnemonic has a 3-way function!
First: **M**onteggia = **U**lna # with **R**adial head **G**one (dislocated)
Second: **M**onteggia = **U**lna #, **R**adial # = **G**aleazzi
Third: **M**onteggia occurs **UP** near the elbow; it's the **R**everse for **G**aleazzi (down near the wrist)

RADIAL HEAD FRACTURE/DISLOCATION

What ligament surrounds the radial head?

The **annular ligament**. It is attached to the radial notch of the **ulna**, but surrounds the radial head *and* neck in the proximal radio-ulnar joint like a pouch

Does it actually attach to radius at all?

No. This allows the radius to rotate freely within it

How do these injuries present?

History: FOOSH
Examination: swelling/ecchymosis at elbow with pain on passive movement. No obvious deformity

Radiology: A **true lat** is very important when assessing the radial head. A **dislocation** will show the radial head is not in alignment with the capitellum [a line drawn through the shaft of the radius (**radiocapitellar line**) should pass through both the radial head and the capitellum].

Always look for ulna #: isolated dislocation is rare!

A fracture of the radial head may be: (i) undisplaced, (ii) displaced, (iii) comminuted (multifragmentary) or (iv) associated with a radial neck fracture. This is a version of **Mason's classification**

Treatment: depends on the injury

Dislocation: if ulna is intact, attempt closed reduction by combination of forced supination of forearm and direct pressure over radial head. AE plaster in supination for 2/52

Undisplaced crack: AE plaster in supination for 4/52

Fragment or through-neck#: K-wire fragment/head to radius and AE plaster in supination for 6/52 and then remove wire

Comminuted #: excise head ±radial head prosthesis; AE plaster in supination for 6/52

What are the complications?

1. **Stiffness** is a common problem in all injuries
2. **OA** of the elbow joint, especially if capitulum cartilage is damaged during injury
3. **Varus deformity** at elbow if radial head is excised (known as **cubitus varus**)

SUPRACONDYLAR FRACTURE OF THE ELBOW

What is this #s claim to fame?

Most common # in kids!

How do they present?

History: FOOSH

Examination: swelling at elbow in tandem with severity of injury; ecchymosis usually present. Pain on passive movement. *Always* check:

1. Pulses as distal blood supply may become compromised (see below)
2. Nerve supply (median, radial and ulnar)

Radiology: severe #s are usually obvious as **transverse** #s of the distal end of the humerus above the condyles, seen best on **lat**. For more subtle ones, **radiocapitellar line** should pass through centre of capitellum on **lat**. Also on **lat,** look for **fat pads** which shows as radiolucent areas around distal end of humerus anteriorly and posteriorly, and signify joint effusion

Anterior fat pad: triangular in shape, may be present normally (syn. **sail sign** due to shape when anterior fat pad lifted off humerus)

Posterior fat pad: *always* abnormal as fat pad significantly displaced out of olecranon fossa; intra-articular pathology *must* be present

Treatment: undisplaced, non-angulated #s can be treated in AE plaster held in angle elbow flexion for 6/52

Displaced/angulated #s may need K-wire fixation if closed reduction fails

Always check pulse/sensation after attempted reduction

What are the complications?

1. **Brachial a. injury**: distal end of humerus usually angulates **posteriorly**, stretching the brachial a. in front, causing spasm or tear, thus compromising blood supply to distal limb
2. **Median n. injury**: the median n. runs medially to the brachial a. at the elbow, and can become stretched during #
3. **Malunion** and **cubitus varus** are possible long-term complications

ELBOW DISLOCATION

How does this injury present?

History: FOOSH with elbow in extension

Examination: obvious deformity at elbow (**S-shaped** deformity). Look at elbow itself: the medial and lateral condyles of the elbow and the olecranon process (the point of the elbow) should form an **equilateral triangle**; this is lost in dislocation

Always assess distal pulses and sensation in median nerve distribution as dislocation has same potential consequences as supracondylar # (see before)

Radiology: dislocation will be obvious; look for associated #s, especially of the **coronoid process** of the ulna, which may cause joint instability, or **radial head #s**

Treatment: in simple dislocation, get assistants to apply traction on forearm and counter-traction on arm while you apply pressure on olecranon process to reduce the dislocation. Treat in sling for 3/52, then mobilise to prevent stiffness

What are the complications?

As with supracondylar # (see before). Avoid passive mobilisation of the elbow as this predisposes to myositis ossificans (heterotropic ossification in the muscles of the elbow) leading to severe stiffness

MID-SHAFT HUMERAL FRACTURE

What must you always be on the look-out for with these #s?

Metastatic bone disease resulting in a **pathological #**

Who usually get this #?

Middle-aged and elderly women

How does it present?

History: FOOSH
Examination: mainly ecchymosis of the arm; deformity may be present. Check **radial nerve** function and sensation
Radiology: # is usually **spiral** (but may be transverse or oblique), and may be displaced or undisplaced. Look carefully for radiolucent areas suggestive of metastatic disease
Treatment: undisplaced #s can be treated in a high AE plaster for 3/52, then changed to brace. Some angulation/displacement is acceptable in humeral #s. Grossly displaced/angulated #s may require ORIF (plating)

What are the complications?

1. **Radial nerve injury**: the radial n. runs in the spiral groove on the posterior aspect of the humerus; damage may cause radial nerve palsy
2. **Mal-/non-union**: this # is notorious for this, and may need ORIF ± bone grafting

SHOULDER DISLOCATION

What main types of shoulder dislocation do you know of?

Anterior and posterior and very rarely inferior (also known as *luxatio erecta*)

Which type is more common?

Anterior (90–95%)

What is the mechanism of injury?

Anterior dislocations are usually caused by trauma, such as **FOOSH**. **Posterior dislocations** are classically caused by the **three Es: electrocution**, **epileptic fit** and **electroconvulsive therapy**, but can also be caused by trauma. **Inferior dislocations** are classically caused by falling down a manhole, with an arm impacting against the sides of the hole

How do anterior dislocations present?

History: FOOSH; may be a Hx of recurrent dislocations causing chronic joint instability

Examination: look for the following:

1. Obvious deformity at shoulder joint (usually a flattening: loss of normal deltoid curve)
2. Adduction and internal rotation of upper limb
3. Acromion process is now most lateral point of shoulder
4. There is axillary fullness due to humeral head's new position
5. Loss of sensation over deltoid area 2ry to axillary n. neuropraxia (**'regiment patch' – UK or 'stars and stripes' area – USA**)
6. Assess pulses distally

Radiology: humeral head is out of glenoid fossa and usually inferior to the coracoid process of the scapula (subcoracoid dislocation); on **lat** the head is anterior to the **Y** that the scapula forms (**golf ball anterior to the tee**). Look for associated #s of glenoid fossa and humeral head/neck

Treatment: in **simple dislocation**, closed reduction under sedation or GA by steady traction of the mildly abducted upper limb with whole-body counter-traction (variation of original **Hippocratic method** – see below). Lying the patient prone with arm hanging over side of bed during traction (**Stimson's method**) may help. **Kocher's method** can also be used (see below) but is associated with an increased risk of fracturing the humeral neck. Treat in body sling for 2–3/52 and then mobilise with physiotherapy. May need open reduction if closed reduction fails

What classic ways of shoulder reduction do you know of?

1. **Kocher's manoeuvre**: involves the following steps:
Mnemonic: **FLAM**
Flex elbow to 90°
Laterally rotate arm 75°
Abduct elbow after lifting it forward
Medially rotate arm
2. **Hippocrates' manoeuvre**: traction is applied to the upper limb while a socked foot applies counter-traction into the axilla where the humeral head lies

What are the complications of anterior dislocation?

1. **Axillary nerve damage** with deltoid weakness/wasting and regiment patch paraesthesia
2. **Axillary artery damage**

3. **# dislocation** needing possible ORIF
4. **Recurrent dislocation**: due to tear of glenoid labrum (lip) ± fracture of glenoid rim causing joint instability; diagnose with MRI and treat with operative stabilisation (eg **Bankart procedure**)

What is the profile of a posterior dislocation?

History: classically an epileptic fit or electrocution, but can be caused by a direct blow to the front of the shoulder

Examination: arm is held in fixed internal rotation; no other gross abnormalities usually detected; pt. is in pain and unwilling to move limb

Radiology: humeral head is usually in glenoid fossa; on **lat** the humeral head assumes a symmetrical shape, like that of a lightbulb (**lightbulb sign**) as opposed to its normal shape which is said to resemble the handle of a walking stick

Treatment: closed reduction by traction and lateral rotation of arm with full-body counter-traction and direct forward pressure of the humeral head from behind. Treat in sling for 2–3/52 with mobilisation and physio after

SURGICAL NECK OF HUMERUS FRACTURE

How many necks does the humerus have?

Two: anatomical and surgical

What is the difference?

The **anatomical neck** is the articular margin of the humeral head. The **surgical neck** is the upper end of the humeral shaft

Which one is more prone to #?

Surgical neck

What lies very close to the surgical neck?

The axillary n.

How does it present?

History: FOOSH
Examination: arm may be held in fixed internal rotation, or may be angulated at the shoulder joint. Ecchymosis
Radiology: # seen; assess angulation, displacement and **impaction** of humeral shaft upwards into humeral head. Also, is humeral head in one piece or many?
Treatment: depends on nature of #:
Impacted #: these are **stable** #s. Can be treated in a collar and cuff for 6/52, followed by physio, as the whole humerus still acts as one piece
Angulated/displaced: if humeral head is whole, but there is angulation/displacement of shaft (humerus acts as 2 pieces), perform closed reduction of shaft (a **hanging slab** applied to distal humerus can be used), and physio in 4–6/52
> 2 pieces: humeral head is not whole and shaft is not impacted: ORIF (plating or hemiarthroplasty, the latter involving replacing the humeral head with a prosthesis)

What are the complications?

1. **Radial nerve damage**: risk of wrist drop
2. **Stiffness** of joint
3. **OA** of shoulder joint later on

PART II

CLAVICULAR FRACTURE/DISLOCATION

What is the clavicle's claim to fame?

It is the first bone in the skeleton to ossify

What is the clavicle's role?

It struts the upper limb (part of the appendicular skeleton) against the trunk (axial skeleton)

Which part of the clavicle usually #s?

The middle third

How does it present?

History: FOOSH.
Examination: there is usually a deformity in the clavicular region with tenting of the overlying skin; the #d end of the proximal segment may or may not pierce the skin
Radiology: # of the middle 1/3 of the clavicle with the distal fragment lying inferiorly to the proximal fragment (sternocleidomastoid pulls proximal fragment superiorly, and the weight of the upper limb pulls the distal fragment inferiorly)
Treatment: conservative management in arm sling for 2/52 then active physio. Any deformity (2ry to **malunion**) is usually accepted

Is there ever place for ORIF?

Not usually, but *may* be considered in:
1. Grossly displaced #s at risk of **non-union**
2. Unacceptable cosmesis
3. Open #s

What is main complication?

Malunion, but again, this is usually accepted

Which end of the clavicle usually dislocates?

The **sternoclavicular joint** (SCJ)

***Where* does it usually dislocate?**

Anteriorly > posteriorly

Which one is more dangerous?

Posterior dislocation, due to potential damage to the adjacent subclavian vessels

How does it present?

History: anterior dislocation can be caused by FOOSH, but is more commonly caused by a direct fall onto the shoulder. Posterior dislocation is caused by direct force to the joint (as in an RTA)

Examination: this will be confined to obvious deformity at the SCJ: anterior = a bulge; posterior = a depression. In posterior dislocation, *assess distal pulses!*

Radiology: diagnosis is usually made clinically, but a **PA oblique view** or a **serendipity view** of the joint will show nature of dislocation

Treatment: non-operative; only compromise to the underlying vessels warrants intervention. Treat in sling and start active physio after 2/52

OTHER MISCELLANEOUS UPPER LIMB FRACTURES

What is a Smith's fracture?

A fracture of the distal end of the radius with **volar** displacement of the distal fragment, caused by a fall onto the back of the wrist

What is it also known as?

A **reverse Colles' fracture**.
Remember, Colles' # involves dorsal displacement of the distal fragment

How is it treated?

With reduction of the fragment (with K-wiring) and AE plaster with the wrist held in **slight extension** for 6/52

PART II

What is a Barton fracture?

A fracture of the distal end of the radius which **involves the radiocarpal joint** (the # line runs *into* the joint, ie is intra-articular). The distal fragment together with the entire carpus are displaced in a volar direction. This # is **unstable** and requires ORIF and plaster for 6/52

What is a Bennett fracture?

An oblique fracture of the base of the 1st metacarpal (ie the thumb metacarpal) extending into the carpometacarpal joint. The distal fragment of the metacarpal is usually displaced. Attempt closed reduction and placing in a **thumb spica**, but K-wiring may be necessary

How are metacarpal #s managed?

Depends on the extent of injury **Minimally or undisplaced**: non-operative; closed reduction and **neighbour/buddy strapping** or BE plaster extending to over *involved* fingers for 3/52 with wrist and hand in safe position (wrist in 20° dorsiflexion, metacarpophalangeal joints at 90° flexion and interphalangeal joints in extension). This safe position holds the ligaments of the respective joints taut so that they do not contract and stiffen with time. Displaced or irreducible: K-wiring/ORIF

What type of #s are MC #s usually?

Mid-shaft

What must be assessed in all MC #s?

Look for rotation of the attached finger(s)

How is this done?	Ask pt. to form a loose fist: all fingers should evenly point towards the **thenar eminence** or **scaphoid**. Deviation from this suggests rotation, and correction should be attempted via closed reduction and neighbour strapping of the affected finger. Rotational status can be confirmed by looking at the fingers end on and ensuring all the nails are aligned evenly
What is a Boxer's fracture?	A fracture of the distal end (head) of the 5th (little finger) metacarpal (usually seen in drunken young men who have punched a wall in anger!)
How are phalangeal #s managed?	Mainly non-operatively with closed reduction where possible and strapping of the broken finger to its neighbour in an attempt to splint it (**neighbour** or **buddy strapping**) for 2–3/52 only. Any longer and stiffness may ensue
What about the distal phalanx?	#s of the distal phalanx are treated as soft tissue injuries. Strapping is not performed. Analgesia, elevation and ice only

HIP FRACTURE AND DISLOCATION

APPLIED ANATOMY

What type of joint is the hip joint?	A synovial, capsulated, ball and socket joint
What is the blood supply to the femoral head?	Three main sources: 1. **Intramedullary aa.** from the femoral shaft

2. **Retinacular aa.** running within the joint capsule, originating from the **medial** and **lateral femoral circumflex aa.** (origin: **profunda femoris**) and running from distal to proximal **Artery of ligamentum teres** (the ligament of the femoral head) (origin: **obturator artery**)

Which one of these is most important?

Depends on the age of the patient. Young patients (kids and young adults) depend on both retinacular and ligamentum teres aa. In older patients, the ligamentum teres a. becomes much less important, and they depend almost entirely on the retinacular supply

What is the surface marking of the femoral head?

The mid-inguinal point: the mid-point of a line drawn from the anterior superior iliac spine (ASIS) to the symphysis pubis. This is also the landmark for the femoral pulse (lies 2 finger-breadths below)

Which ligaments stabilise the hip joint?

Three in all:
1. **Iliofemoral** ligament (of Bigelow): the strongest and is described as being 'Y-shaped'
2. **Pubofemoral** ligament
3. **Ischiofemoral** ligament (Easily remembered as each ligament arises from each of the 3 bony components of the acetabulum; see above)

From where does the hip capsule arise?

The labrum of the acetabulum and the transverse ligament (which bridges the acetabular notch)

Where does it attach?	The femoral neck. Anteriorly, it attaches to the intertrochanteric line. Posteriorly, it attaches to the neck, but only up to half the distance of the anterior attachment

HIP FRACTURE

How can hip #s be broadly classified?	As **intracapsular** and **extracapsular** fractures
What's the difference?	**Intracapsular #s** occur *within* the hip joint capsule. **Extracapsular #s** occur outside the capsule, usually between the greater and lesser trochanters of the femur (but can also occur distal to them)
What are extracapsular #s therefore also known as?	As **intertrochanteric #s**, as these are the most common type. **Subtrochanteric #s** are far less common and are often pathological, eg secondary to bone metastases
What is the clinical significance of this?	In **intracapsular #s**, the retinacular blood supply to the femoral head is disturbed, therefore rendering it at risk of **avascular necrosis**. In **intertrochanteric #s**, the femoral head's blood supply is *not* affected. Treatment of each type of # is therefore different
How can intracapsular #s be further classified?	By the use of **Garden's classification**. This classification unfortunately does not help with treatment or prognosis; it is better to divide intracapsular fractures into undisplaced (Grades 1 and 2 or Garden's) or displaced (3 and 4)

PART II

What is Garden's classification?

A classification of the severity of intracapsular #s based on the integrity of the trabeculae on AP film (see Figure 5.1)

Figure 5.1

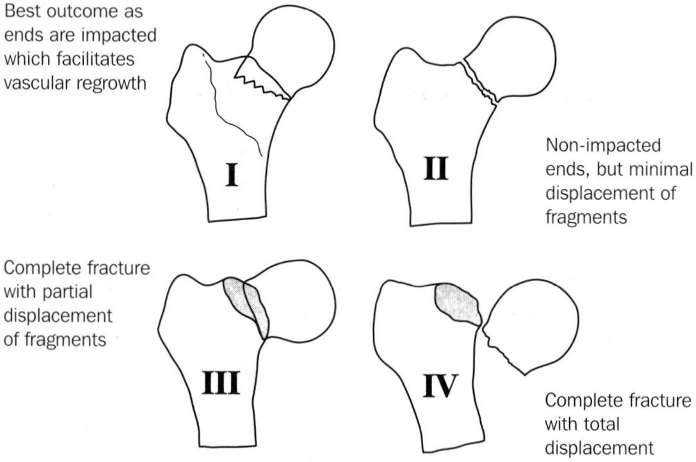

Best outcome as ends are impacted which facilitates vascular regrowth

Non-impacted ends, but minimal displacement of fragments

Complete fracture with partial displacement of fragments

Complete fracture with total displacement

Who usually gets hip #s?

The elderly, but especially women because of weaker bones 2ry to **osteoporosis**

How do they present?

History: Following a fall, usually mechanical, but may be non-mechanical (eg following dizziness, TIA, etc)

Examination: Shortened, rotated (usually externally) lower limb upon which weight cannot be borne. Always check for pulses and sensation distally

If asked about what fractures are important to consider when treating hip fractures, consider the **four Ms**: **mechanical/non-mechanical fall**, pre-injury **mobility**, **morbidity** (ie what other medical conditions does the patient have) and **mental state** (what is their mini-mental test score?)

What are the investigations?

Blood investigations: routine investigations, but also a GXM 2 U
Imaging: AP/lat hip X-ray
Other: investigation of cause of fall in non-mechanical cases (may need medical referral)

What is the difference in management of the two types of hip #s?

Broadly speaking, **intracapsular #s** need excision of the femoral head and insertion of a metal prosthesis (**hemiarthroplasty**) – a **head-replacing** procedure
Extracapsular #s are treated by ORIF of the femoral head to the neck using cannulated screws – a **head-preserving** procedure
Mnemonic: In Garden's classification, 1, 2 try and screw; 3, 4 throw the head out the door!
Extracapsular #s are treated with ORIF, usually in the form of a **dynamic hip screw** (DHS) *without* excision of the femoral head

PART II

HIP DISLOCATION

What types of hip dislocations do you know of?

Anterior and posterior

Which one is more common?

Posterior (90–95%) – the opposite of shoulder dislocations)

How does it occur?	Usually following RTAs, but sometimes due to fall. Can also occur following hip replacements
What are the complications?	1. Sciatic nerve damage due to pressure by the dislocated head; may cause a foot drop 2. Acetabular fracture 3. AVN of femoral head due to disruption of blood supply 4. Secondary OA
What are the important points in the history?	1. How did the incident occur? 2. If RTA, what damage did the vehicle sustain? 3. Any knee injuries (knee-to-dashboard injury during RTA is a very common cause of posterior hip dislocation)? 4. Any other associated injuries?
What are the clinical findings?	The limb is shortened, adducted and internally rotated (posterior dislocation). Look for knee injury/deformity and foot drop
What is the management?	1. Analgesia 2. Imaging: AP/lat hip joint **and** knee 3. Reduce under sedation/GA; assess for stability at the same time, and apply traction (either skeletal in the form of a pin through the tibia, or skin). Reduce the joint as soon as possible, as delay to reduction (especially over 6 hours) is associated with an increased risk of AVN
What should be done next?	Obtain a CT scan. If #d acetabulum or unacceptable reduction, operative intervention is required

LOWER LIMB FRACTURES

Note: The hip # is technically a lower limb #, but, because of its importance and the frequency with which you are likely to encounter it during your rotation, it has been dealt with separately in Section C above.

What main lower limb #s do you know of?

The following:
Femur:
1. Hip (femoral neck) (see 'Hip fracture and dislocation' above)
2. Mid-shaft

Knee:
1. Supracondylar femoral
2. Patellar
3. Tibial plateau and condylar

Tibia/fibula (tib-fib):
1. Mid-shaft

Ankle:
1. Ankle mortise #s

FEMORAL SHAFT FRACTURE

What are the main types of femoral shaft #s?

Mid-shaft and supracondylar

What are femoral supracondylar #s claim to fame?

They are the most common #s occurring around the knee

Profile of mid-shaft #s?

History: direct trauma (RTA), twisting injuries in sports, heavy falls. Pathological #s also occur (usually in elderly due to secondary deposit)
Examination: look for signs of shock. The limb is usually swollen and deformed. Assess for open wound, and neurovascular status distally. Examine for other associated injuries
Radiology: shows #

Management: treat shock if present (ABCs). If open wound present, cover with Betadine®-soaked swab. Give analgesia. Splint limb and apply distal skin traction. ORIF (IMN or plate and screws) if closed; Ex-Fix if open

How do they present?

History: Usually a fall in an elderly patient

Examination: Swelling, ecchymosis and deformity around the knee. Assess distal neurovascular status

Radiology: shows #; assess degree of angulation and look for other #s

Management: place in AK slab. ORIF is usually needed

What are the possible complications of femoral #s?

1. Shock
2. Fat embolism
3. Non-union
4. Delayed union
5. Malunion
6. Neurological (sciatic nerve)
7. Vascular compromise (esp. popliteal a.)

PATELLAR FRACTURE AND DISLOCATION

What attaches to the patella?

The quadriceps tendon at the superior pole and the patellar ligament at the inferior pole. The patellar ligament also attaches to the tibial tuberosity. The three act together to raise (extend) the leg during quadriceps contraction

How do #s present?

History: direct fall onto the knee, with resulting inability to straight leg raise

Examination: swelling and ecchymosis around the knee. Crepitus may be palpable. There may be an inability to straight leg raise

Radiology: determine whether # is transverse (most common), longitudinal or comminuted
Treatment: depends on the type
Transverse: ORIF (eg with tension band wiring) as continuity of straight-leg-raising mechanism is disturbed
Longitudinal/comminuted: non-operated in long leg cylinder cast for 6–8/52

What are the complications?

1. Knee stiffness
2. Delayed/non-union
3. Complex regional pain syndrome (rare)

How do dislocations present?

History: twisting injury of knee, more commonly in young girls (see below)
Examination: deformed knee ± swelling (depends on concurrent ligamentous injury) with knee in a mildly flexed position. Patella is usually laterally displaced
Radiology: confirms dislocation; r/o #s
Treatment: reduction under sedation: apply pressure to patella in direction opposite to dislocation whilst extending knew

What stabilises the patella and prevents lateral dislocation?

Three components:
Bony, eg lateral femoral condyle
Ligamentous, eg medial retinacular fibres
Muscular, eg pull of vastus medialis

TIBIAL PLATEAU FRACTURE

What are these?

Fractures involving the proximal (upper) end of the tibia and its articular surface

Which one is more common?

Tibial plateau #

PART II

79

Of the tibial plateaux, which one is more commonly #d?

The lateral tibial plateau

How do these present?

History: RTA and falls (usually off horse or bike)

Examination: pain, ecchymosis and swelling around knee. Deformity is not usually a feature

Radiology: assess whether plateau, condyle or both are involved. Isolated tibial plateau #s may be difficult to assess on plain film. CT is usually needed to assess full extent

Treatment: depends on the #. Because upper end of tibia is composed of easily compressed cancellous bone, a bone graft is sometimes needed to strut fragments to normal positions and restore joint congruity

Plateau: ORIF (plate and screws), usually with bone graft to strut plateau fragment and regain articular continuity

Condyle: ORIF (plate and screws) ± bone graft

What are the complications?

1. Delayed/non-/malunion
2. Post-traumatic arthritis (articular involvement)

TIBIAL-FIBULAR (TIB-FIB) FRACTURES

What are tib-fib #s claim to fame?

High incidence of compound (open) #s requiring external fixation; wound infection with resulting osteomyelitis; and union problems (delayed, mal- and non-union)

How do they present?

History: sporting injury, fall or RTA. Isolated fibular #s usually occur secondary to a direct blow

Examination: leg may be deformed with bony fragment protruding from skin (open #). Swelling and ecchymosis. Assess distal neurovascular status

Radiology: assess # for displacement, angulation and for which of the bones is #d (tibia, fibula or both?)

Treatment: if # is **closed**, ORIF (IMN or plates/screws) may be undertaken if displaced or angulated. If undisplaced, non-operative management in AK plaster for 8/52 may suffice

If **open**, thorough washout and debridement of the wound is necessary, followed by application of an Ex-Fix or IMN

What increases the chance of union problems?

If the tibia is fractured in isolation. The intact fibula acts as a strut, keeping the ends of the tibial # apart

ANKLE MORTISE FRACTURES

What is the ankle mortise?

The area made up of the following:
1. Distal articular surface of the tibia
2. Medial malleolus
3. Lateral malleolus
4. Posterior malleolus
5. Talus

What are the malleoli?

The **medial malleolus** is the distal tibial condyle

The **lateral malleolus** is the distal end of the fibula

There is also a **posterior malleolus**, which is the posterior part of the distal end of the tibia

What stabilises the ankle mortise?

The **distal tibiofibular syndesmosis**, which is made up of the following:

1. Anterior and posterior tibiofibular ligaments
2. Inferior transverse ligament
3. Interosseous ligament

How stable are ankle #s?

Depends mainly on how many malleoli are #d during the injury. Bi- and tri-malleolar #s are usually highly unstable and require ORIF

How do they present?

History: usually a twisting injury, commonly during sports. Ask whether injury involved inversion or eversion of the foot (will clue in on what type of # to expect)

Examination: gross swelling and ecchymosis of the ankle with associated deformity

Radiology: assess the malleoli and how many are #d (look closely for **avulsion #s** as well, which may represent severe ligamentous injury and may be just as unstable as full-blown #s). Look for **talar shift**: talus may be grossly or mildly displaced within the mortise; even mild shift is a sign of ankle instability. In isolated medial malleolar #, *do AP/lat of knee*, as fibula may # at its neck instead of at its distal (lateral malleolar) end, and may be missed. This high fibular fracture is known as a **Maisonneuve's fracture**

Treatment: usually depends on number of malleoli #d, degree of talar shift and displacement of fragments. Generally, most unstable ankle #s will need ORIF (plate and screws)

Non-operative management in BK plaster cast for 6–8/52 is reserved for stable (usually unimalleolar), undisplaced #s

What are the complications?

1. Delayed/non-/malunion
2. Post-traumatic arthritis (articular involvement)

What is the risk from fibular neck #?

Damage to the common peroneal n. which wraps round it. May present as lateral foot paraesthesia or as a full-blown foot drop

OTHER MISCELLANEOUS LOWER LIMB FRACTURES

What makes talar #s complicated?

The complex anatomy of the bone and its blood supply

How is it #d?

Secondary to high energy trauma

Is it common?

No, it is rare

What are the findings?

Severe swelling and pain of the foot

What is the management?

X-rays, and BK plaster if undisplaced. If displaced, ORIF. CT scan may be necessary

What are the complications?

1. **Avascular necrosis**
2. Mal-/nonunion
3. Ankle stiffness

What makes calcaneal #s complicated?

They also have a complex anatomy and blood supply

How is it #d?

Fall from a height

Is it common?

Yes, relatively

What are the findings?

Severe swelling and pain of the heel/foot. Examine back as well, as if fall was from very high, there may be associated vertebral crush #s

Radiology?

Plain film ±CT scan of heel, and plain films of spine

PART II

Treatment?	Most surgeons advocate conservative treatment in BK plaster. Some perform ORIF (plate and screws). This is a controversial area of orthopaedics
Complications?	Sub-talar stiffness and arthritis
Are metatarsal #s common?	Yes
How do they occur?	Inversion injuries of the foot
Which one is most commonly #d?	The 5th metatarsal
How are they managed?	Either with strapping or BK plaster (boot). ORIF is rarely needed
What about phalangeal #s?	Usually caused by stubbing of the toe. Treat conservatively by strapping of the toe. Occasionally K-wiring may be necessary, especially in big toe #s

TENDINOUS, LIGAMENTOUS AND MENISCAL INJURIES

MENISCAL INJURY

What are the menisci?	Crescent-shaped cartilaginous structures situated between the tibial plateau and the medial and lateral femoral condyles. There are 2 menisci: medial and lateral (singular: meniscus).
Which one is more commonly injured?	The medial meniscus
What is the usual nature of the injury?	A twisting injury of the knee, usually sport related (especially football and rugby)
How does it present?	1. Pain over the inner (or outer if lateral) aspect of the knee 2. Swelling 3. **Locking** (almost pathognomonic) 4. 'Giving way' of the knee

What causes locking?	A torn bit of meniscus getting caught between the femoral condyle and the tibial plateau during movement of the joint
What are the examination findings?	1. Swelling 2. May present with a locked knee 3. Tender joint line on palpation (a transverse line drawn through the joint space between the distal end of the femur and the proximal end of the tibia), either medially or laterally depending on which meniscus is involved 4. Positive McMurray's test
What is McMurray's test?	Forced flexion and external rotation of the knee combined with medial compression of the medial joint line elicits pain in medial meniscal injury Lateral meniscus tested by reversing the test (internal rotation and lateral compression)
How are meniscal injuries investigated?	MRI of the knee
How are they treated?	Arthroscopic trimming of the tear and, occasionally, repair

LIGAMENTOUS KNEE INJURY

What are the main ligaments of the knee?	The medial and lateral **collateral ligaments** and the anterior and posterior **cruciate ligaments**
How do they afford stability to the knee?	**Collaterals**: occur on either side of the knee and limit valgus and varus movement of the joint

PART II

Cruciates: occur within the joint, crossing each other (hence *cruciate* or cross-like), and limiting anterior (anterior cruciate) and posterior (posterior cruciate) translation of the tibia

Which ligament is most commonly injured?

The medial collateral ligament

How is it damaged?

Usually due to **valgus strain** at the knee, a common sport injury

What are the symptoms?

Pain and swelling ± instability

What are the examination findings?

Pain on valgus strain, with opening up of joint laterally in complete rupture

What other injuries may be associated with it?

The 3 following knee injuries are oftentimes found together:
1. Medial collateral ligament injury
2. Medial meniscal tear
3. Anterior cruciate ligament tear/rupture

Also known as **O'Donohue's triad**

What are the symptoms of anterior cruciate ligament (ACL) rupture?

Pain, inability to weight bear and almost immediate swelling due to haemarthrosis (bleeding into the joint)

What are the examination findings?

Pain, swelling and ecchymosis (due to haemarthrosis)
Lachman test is positive (with pt. lying down with knee flexed, tibia can be drawn forward in relation to the femur due to ACL laxity). As is the anterior drawer test (similar to Lachman's but with the knee flexed to 90°

What imaging is necessary?

MRI of the knee. A plain film should also be done to r/o bony injury

| What is the treatment of ACL rupture? | Non-operative treatment if stable knee and low-demand patient; ACL reconstruction (ACLR) for unstable knee and high-demand patient. Physio is vital for rehabilitation |

ACHILLES' TENDON RUPTURE

What is the Achilles' tendon?	The tendon of the gastrocnemius (calf muscle)
Where is it attached to?	The posterior aspect of the calcaneus (heel bone)
What is its function?	Plantar flexion
How is it ruptured?	By missing a step (esp. during dancing), running or during sport (especially tennis). Steroids and use of fluoroquinolone antibiotics (especially ciprofloxacin) ↑ risk
What does the patient notice?	Typically a sharp 'snapping sensation' followed by an immediate inability to weight bear on that leg
What are the clinical findings?	An obvious gap in the tendon just above the heel which may be seen and felt (have the patient lie prone or kneel on a chair) There is a failure of the foot to plantar flex on squeezing the calf (**Simmond's** or **Thompson's** test)
What is the treatment?	May be non-operative or operative **Non-operative**: AK plaster with foot in equinus position [exaggerated plantar flexion like a horse's (hence *equinus*) hoof] for 4–6/52. Can change to removable walking brace for further 4/52 **Operative**: primary repair of tendon and plaster in equinus for 4–6/52

PART II

| When do you use which? | Largely depends on wishes and physical demands of patient and preference of surgeon. Outcomes are generally similar but risk of re-rupture is less with surgical repair |

ANKLE SPRAIN

Which ligament is most commonly injured?	The lateral ligament complex
What type of injury is it?	Usually an inversion injury
What are the symptoms?	Pain, swelling (not usually nearly as much as is seen in an ankle #, unless an avulsion # is associated) and ecchymosis. Deformity is not a feature, though instability may be present
Imaging?	If diagnosis is uncertain, perform AP/lat to r/o #
How is it managed?	**Simple sprain**: RICE (rest, ice, compression, elevation) and then mobilise **Ligamentous tear**: ankle support and physiotherapy **Symptomatic instability**: surgical stabilisation

COMPARTMENT SYNDROME

What is compartment syndrome?

It comprises the following events:
↑ pressure in the fascial compartments of the limb secondary to oedema (in this case)
↓
↓ venous outflow
↓
further ↑ in intra-compartmental pressure
↓
compromised arterial inflow
↓
muscle ischaemia and necrosis

What are the causes?

1. Fractures: most common lower limb cause is a tibial #; in the upper limb, injuries around the elbow and forearm
2. Crush injury
3. Burns
4. Snake bite
5. Prolonged surgical procedure (esp. lithotomy position)

What are the signs?

The **6 Ps**:
Pain
Paraesthesia (late)
Paralysis (late)
Pallor (late)
Perishingly cold (late)
Pulselessness (very late)

What is the most important of these?

Pain, specifically:
Pain out of proportion with the history
Pain on passive stretching of affected muscles
Pain on palpation of affected muscle groups

PART II

What can be used to clinically assess it?

A hand-held device specifically designed for the purpose. If pressure is >30 mmHg or if the measured pressure is within 30 mmHg of the diastolic pressure, compartment syndrome is likely and **immediate fasciotomy** (or escharotomy in the case of circumferential burns; see Chapter 10) is required

What does a fasciotomy entail?

Division of the fascia enclosing the involved muscular compartment via a surgical incision, causing a release in pressure. In the lower leg, the anterior, lateral, superficial posterior and deep posterior fascial compartments must all be released

What about the use of a Doppler USS?

Not clinically useful as it can detect a waveform at very low pulse pressures and may give false reassurance

Does a weak or absent pulse automatically mean compartment syndrome?

Not necessarily. Weak or absent pulses *may* be due to compartment syndrome but consider underfilling and vascular injury in your differential. The signs outlined above are more indicative

CHAPTER 6: GENERAL ORTHOPAEDICS

OSTEOARTHRITIS (OA)

What is osteoarthritis?

A non-inflammatory degenerative joint disease characterised by progressive loss of articular cartilage with associated new bone formation and capsular fibrosis

What causes it?

Failure of chondrocytes to repair damaged cartilage (wear > repair) or primary damage to cartilage

How is it classified?

Primary: no obvious cause
Secondary: previous trauma, limb deformity, obesity, infection, metabolic disorder

Who gets it?

80–90% of people > 65 years have evidence of 1ry OA. F>M (up to 12:1 in knee OA)

What are the symptoms?

May be asymptomatic for years, only being noticeable in old age:
1. Stiffness which gradually worsens as the day progresses [as opposed to morning stiffness in rheumatoid arthritis (RA) secondary to inflammatory exudates that build up overnight] gradual worsening
2. Joint pain
3. Reduced range of motion
4. Joint crepitus

What is found on examination?

May be normal clinically. The joint may be stiff and range of movement ↓. **Heberden's nodes** may be present in the hands (palpable swellings in DIPJs representing osteophytes)

What are the radiological findings?

Always say the following (**LOSS**):
1. **L**oss of joint space
2. **O**steophytes
3. **S**ubchondral sclerosis
4. **S**ubchondral cysts

What is an osteophyte?

An irregular outgrowth of new bone (the bone's attempt at regenerating the bone lost to **wear and tear** is done in a haphazard fashion)

What is a joint mouse?

An osteophyte which breaks off into the intra-articular space as a loose body

What is the management?

Non-operative and operative.
Non-operative:
1. Avoid excessive strain on joint: **lose weight**, avoid high impact activity
2. Physiotherapy (maintain range of joint motion)
3. NSAIDs (eg diclofenac) or COX-2 inhibitors (eg parecoxib)
4. Intra-articular steroid injections (during inflammatory flare-ups)
5. Intra-articular viscosupplementation (eg hyaluronic acid)
6. Oral viscosupplementation (eg chondroitin, glucosamine)

Operative:
1. **Arthroscopy** (for debridement and wash-out) may be helpful
2. **Osteotomy** to realign the involved joint
3. Total prosthetic joint replacement (**arthroplasty**)
4. **Arthrodesis** (fusion) in selected patients

These four operations are the four options for surgical treatment of joint disorders in orthopaedics!

SEPTIC ARTHRITIS

What types of arthritis related to infection do you know of?

Septic and reactive.
Septic arthritis: direct invasion of the joint space by infection (direct inoculation, spread from bloodstream or from infected peri-articular tissue or prosthesis)
Reactive arthritis: a sterile inflammatory process secondary to an infective process somewhere else in the body

What organisms cause these conditions?

Septic arthritis: bacterial infections are by far most common, though mycobacteria, viruses and fungi may also cause it.
1. *Staphylococcus aureus*: most common pathogen in patients over the age of 2
2. *Neisseria gonorrhoea*: most common pathogen in young, sexually active adults
3. Gram –ve bugs are found in the very young and very old

Reactive arthritis: common in patients who are HLA-B27 positive, and have GI problems (eg UC/Crohn's). Responsible bugs include:
1. *Salmonella enteritidis*
2. *Salmonella typhimurium*
3. *Yersinia enterocolitica*
4. *Campylobacter jejuni*
5. *Clostridium difficile*
6. *Shigella sonnei*
7. *Entamoeba histolytica*
8. *Cryptosporidium*

Other causes include UTI 2ry to *Chlamydia trachomatis*

PART II

What are the important points in the history?

1. Onset: acute or chronic?
2. Mono- or polyarticular?
3. Injury to joint, or recent surgery (incl. arthroscopy)?
4. Extra-articular symptoms (suggest systemic disease/reactive arthritis)?
5. Intravenous drug abuse?
6. STD?
7. Immunocompromised state (eg AIDS, immunosuppressive drugs)?
8. Underlying joint disease (eg rheumatoid arthritis, gout)?

What is the hallmark sign of septic arthritis?

Inability to move joint *at all*

What other signs are present?

General: pyrexial ± rigors. Signs of systemic disease may be present
Joint: red, swollen, tender, minimal movement

What are the investigations?

Blood investigations:
1. FBC: ↑WBC
2. CRP: raised
3. Urate: may be raised in gout
4. ESR: raised
5. Blood cultures: r/o bacteraemia as cause

Radiology: plain film to r/o underlying joint disease and osteomyelitis

Other: A joint aspiration *must* be done under sterile conditions. Send fluid off for:
1. M/C/S
2. Urgent Gram stain
3. Crystals

What is the management?

1. Admit
2. IV fluids
3. IV antibiotics; change pending M/C/S results

4. Elevate limb and splint for comfort if necessary
5. Book for arthroscopic wash-out of joint

BONY TUMOURS

What types of benign bony tumours do you know of?

See Table 6.1

Table 6.1

	Osteoma	Chondroma	Osteochondroma	Giant-cell tumour
Appearance/ Radiology	Smooth, rounded prominence on long, flat or skull bone	Tumour may grow from the bone (ecchondroma) or within the bone, expanding it (enchondroma). Common in the hands and feet	Mushroom-like growth starting at epiphyseal plate in kids, but migrating towards shaft as bone grows	Lower femur or upper tibia. Radiolucent area seen on X-ray with expansion of cortex
Composition/ Pathology	Either hard, compact bone (**ivory osteoma**) or cancellous bone	Cartilaginous	Bony core, capped by cartilage	Destruction of bone substance with formation of new sub-periosteal bone
Symptoms	Palpable swelling	Palpable swelling	Palpable swelling, usually near a joint	Pain and swelling
Treatment	Simple excision	No treatment unless unsightly	Excision	Wide local excision ± bone graft and/or prosthesis
Other	**Osteoid osteomas** are benign bone tumours of unknown aetiology that classically present with pain relieved by NSAIDs and appear radiologically as a small sclerotic bone island (nidus) with a circular lucent defect	Prone to pathological #. May give rise to chondrosarcoma	Most common benign bony tumour	Syn. **osteoclastoma.** Though benign, may metastasise. Pathological # common

What is the most common type of bone cancer?

Trick question. The answer is **bony metastasis**, or secondary bone tumour. Primary bone tumours are *uncommon*

What tumours metastasise to bone?

Mnemonic:
Bony **P**ain = **L**ikely **K**iller **T**umour
Breast
Prostate
Lung
Kidney
Thyroid
In order of decreasing frequency

What is a pathological #?

A # which occurs through an area of bony weakness caused by an underlying bony tumour (benign or, more commonly, malignant) or other condition, eg metabolic bone disease such as osteoporosis

What type of primary malignant tumours do you know of?

See Table 6.2

Table 6.2

	Osteosarcoma	Chondrosarcoma	Ewing's tumour	Multiple myeloma
Occurrence	Childhood and adolescence	Middle aged	Children	Middle aged and older
Site	Lower femur, upper tibia, upper humerus	Femur, tibia, humerus (central) or flat bones (peripheral)	Femoral shaft, tibia and humerus	Skeleton-wide with multiple lesions present
Pathology	Arises from primitive bone-forming cells, destroying bone structure. Mainly fibrous. May occur 2ry to Paget's disease of bone	Arises from cartilage cells, either *de novo* or from a chondroma	Endothelial sarcoma of bone, arising from endothelial elements in marrow. A soft, vascular tumour	Bone plasma-cell origin. **Bence–Jones protein** found in urine. Marrow biopsy shows plasma-cell proliferation
Clinical features	Pain and swelling	Pain and swelling; may grow to very large size	Pain and swelling, usually midshaft	General ill-health and microcytic anaemia. Local bone pain and swelling

Table 6.2 *Continued*

	Osteosarcoma	Chondrosarcoma	Ewing's tumour	Multiple myeloma
Radiology	Metaphyseal destruction. New sub-periosteal bone formation (**Codman's triangle**) Radiating new-bone spicule formation (**sun-burst appearance**)	Soft-tissue shadow either growing from bone surface (peripheral) or bursting through cortex (central)	Bone destruction with concentric layers of new subperiosteal bone (**onion-skinning appearance**)	Multiple small, well-circumscribed radio-lucent areas. Pathological #s common
Treatment	Chemotherapy + surgical excision ± prosthesis ± amputation	Wide surgical excision ± prosthesis ± amputation	Chemotherapy + operative excision with prosthesis. Radiotherapy in upper limb and pelvis	Chemotherapy. Local radiotherapy for bony foci
Prognosis	Improved since chemo; lung mets common	Good as slow growing and few mets	Used to be fatal; chemo has improved to 50–60% at 5 years. Mets common	Often fatal

Can tumour site clue in to the type of tumour present?

Yes. See Table 6.3

Table 6.3

Site	Typical tumour found
Epiphyseal	Chondroblastoma Aneurysmal bone cyst Giant cell tumour
Metaphyseal	Any lesion
Diaphyseal	Osteoblastoma Lymphoma Fibrous dysplasia
Pelvis	Metastatic disease Multiple myeloma Ewing's sarcoma Paget's disease
Proximal humerus	Chondroid lesions

Continued

Table 6.3 *Continued*

Site	Typical tumour found
Knee	Osteosarcoma Chondromyxoid fibroma
Ribs	Metastatic disease Multiple myeloma Ewing's sarcoma Fibrous dysplasia
Spine	**Vertebral body**: Metastatic disease Multiple myeloma Chondroma Paget's disease Haemangioma
	Posterior elements: Aneurysmal bone cyst Osteoid osteoma Osteoblastoma
Periosteal	Osteosarcoma Chondrosarcoma Chondroma
Multiple lesions	Metastatic disease Multiple myeloma Haemangioma Fibrous dysplasia Osteochondromas Histiocytosis X (Langerhan's cell histiocytosis)

What is the most common primary bone tumour?   Osteosarcoma

PAEDIATRIC ORTHOPAEDICS

GENERAL

Define the following:

Epiphysis	The end of a long bone
Physis	The cartilaginous growth area of bone
Metaphysis	The shaft of a long bone
What is a greenstick #?	A fracture in which one side (the tension side) of a bone is broken while the other (the compression side) is bent (like a green stick)
What is a plastic bowing #?	A fracture where a long bone is bent but not actually broken. It is a prelude to the greenstick # because if the bone continues to bend, one side (the tension side) will eventually break
What is a torus #?	A fracture in which the cortex buckles due to an axial load. Also known as a buckle fracture
How are paediatric #s involving the physis classified?	By using the **Salter–Harris** classification (I-V) (See Figure 6.1)

Figure 6.1

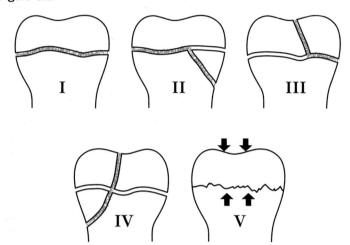

How can it be remembered?	*Mnemonic:* SALTeR
	I: **S**eparation
	II: **A**bove (through metaphysis)
	III: **L**ower than (through epiphysis)
	IV: **T**hrough (metaphysic and epiphysis)
	V: **R**educed or **R**ammed (compression injury)

What is the order of ossification centres around the elbow?	*Mnemonic:*
	Come **R**ide **M**y **T**ool **O**f **L**ove
	Capitellum — 1 year
	Radial head — 3 years
	Medial epicondyle — 5 years
	Trochlea — 7 years
	Olecranon — 9 years
	Lateral epicondyle — 11 years

DEVELOPMENTAL DYSPLASIA OF THE HIP (DDH)

What is it?

A spectrum of developmental disorders of the hip ranging from acetabular dysplasia to dislocation
Incidence is 1 in 1000

Who gets it?

Mnemonic: **All the Fs**
F:M = 7:1
The following increase incidence:
1. Breech delivery (**F**aulty position)
2. **First born** ($\downarrow$ intrauterine space)
3. Oligohydramnios ($\downarrow$ liquor volume – **F**luid problems)
4. **F**amily history

Describe some common abnormalities?

Excessive capsular laxity and a shallow acetabulum at birth may be present

How does it present?

Either at birth (picked up on routine exam) or at a few months of age as a dislocated hip (shortening and decreased abduction). Limp may be present if picked up late or a waddling gait if bilateral

What are the clinical findings?

Obvious deformity may be visible. There may be **asymmetry of groin crease**, especially if an extra posterior perineal crease. Perform the following tests:
Barlow's test: hip is flexed and thigh adducted, while pushing posteriorly in line of the shaft of femur, causing femoral head to dislocate posteriorly from acetabulum. Dislocation is palpable as femoral head slips out of acetabulum
Ortolani's test:
1. Infant's legs placed in frog-leg position
2. Place middle finger on greater trochanter

3. Use thumb and index finger to hold knee
4. Attempt relocation of femoral head into acetabulum by pushing upwards (away from bed) on greater trochanter

Interpretation: if a **clunk** is felt, this means the femoral head has relocated back into acetabulum, suggesting a reducible hip

What is the investigation of choice?

Ultrasound of the hip joint when less than 6 months and plain pelvic radiograph if older

How is it managed?

Depends on age:
< 6 months: Pavlik harness until reduction confirmed and hip developing normally. If unsuccessful, for open reduction at 6/12 age
6–18 months: Closed ± open reduction ± femoral osteotomy
> 18 months: open reduction ± femoral and pelvic osteotomy

PERTHES' DISEASE

What is Perthes' disease?

Idiopathic osteonecrosis of the epiphysis of the femoral head, causing collapse and deformity. Incidence is 1 in 10,000

What is the outcome?

Osteoarthritis in later life

Who gets it?

Male children; M:F = 5:1. More common in whites

What is the history?

Groin pain, referred knee pain, limp. No trauma usually reported

What are the clinical findings?

Shortened lower limb; antalgic (painful) gait, muscle spasm and wasting (2ry to disuse) with unwillingness to have limb moved

What is seen on radiology?	Deformed femoral head clinches diagnosis. Technetium scan can detect avascular necrotic changes at early stage in disease before X-ray findings are evident. MRI can also be used
How is it treated?	By maintaining the femoral head within the acetabulum (containment) while preserving range of motion. Most often treated non-operatively but occasionally surgery required for containment or for deformity

SLIPPED UPPER FEMORAL EPIPHYSIS (SUFE)

What is SUFE?	The upper femoral epiphysis slips and becomes abnormally placed in relation to the femoral neck Incidence is 1 in 100,000
What direction does the epiphysis slip?	Inferiorly and posteriorly in relation to the femoral neck (although strictly the epiphysis stays in its place and it's the femoral neck that moves)
Who gets it?	Adolescents. M:F = 2.5:1. More common in blacks
What makes one more prone to it?	Hormonal problems (especially in young children) Look for: **Fröhlich's syndrome**: short and fat (GH normal, $\downarrow$ sex hormones) **Marfanoid build**: tall and thin (GH $\uparrow$, sex hormones normal) Panhypopituitarism and hypothyroidism may be also associated
What are the symptoms?	Antalgic gait, groin pain, referred knee pain
What are the investigations?	AP/lat hip X-rays confirm the diagnosis

What is the management? Operative: depends on whether slip is mild or severe. Anything from threaded screws to complex osteotomies may be indicated to restore pre-slip angle of epiphysis in relation to the femoral neck

CONGENITAL TALIPES EQUINOVARUS (CTEV)

What is it commonly known as? Club foot

What causes it? Aetiology unknown

What is its incidence? 1:1000 live births

What does the foot look like? The forefoot is adducted and supinated; the hind foot is inverted and plantar flexed (in equinus). There may also be cavus (arched sole) There may also be **prominent creases** due to contracture of fascial planes beneath the skin

What are the important points in the history? The following questions should be asked:
1. Is there a generalised abnormality?
2. Is the spine normal?
3. Is there abnormal joint laxity?
4. Are there constriction bands?

Can it be detected *in utero*? Yes, via ultrasound during the 2nd trimester

How is it treated? Either non-operatively or operatively
Non-operative: start immediately after birth. Serial casting (change every 1–2/52 until correction) using the revolutionary Ponseti technique
Surgical: involves soft tissue release, tendon transfers and/or osteotomy to correct deformity, progressing to correction with external fixators (Ilizarov technique) and arthrodesis for recurrences and in later life

PART III

The subspecialties

CHAPTER 7: PAEDIATRIC SURGERY

THORAX

TRACHEO-OESOPHAGEAL FISTULAE (TOF)

What is a TOF?
A congenital or acquired abnormal communication between the trachea and the oesophagus

Which type is more common?
Congenital TOF

What is the UK frequency?
1:3500 live births

What causes it?
No definite cause exists

What types of congenital TOF do you know of?
1. Oesophageal atresia with distal TOF
2. Isolated TOF
3. Oesophageal atresia with proximal TOF
4. Oesophageal atresia with proximal and distal TOF (H-type)

(See Figure 7.1)

Figure 7.1

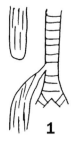 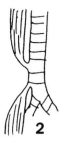 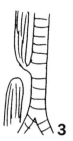 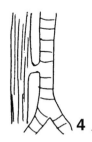

1   2   3   4

What other congenital abnormalities may occur?
The oesophagus may also be atretic *without* any TOF present. The mid-oesophagus may also be absent

Which one is most common?
Oesophageal atresia with distal TOF (85%)

When do congenital TOFs present?

At birth or during the 1st year of life

When should TOF be looked out for?

In a woman who develops **polyhydramnios** [high liquor (pronounced *lie*-kor) volume] during pregnancy

How does TOF present?

1. Fine frothy secretions at the mouth which recur during suctioning
2. Noisy breathing with coughing/ choking spells associated with **apnoea**
3. Symptoms which **worsen during feeding** (feed entering respiratory tract)

Does TOF present as an isolated abnormality?

It *can*, but many occur with other developmental abnormalities (up to 70%):

1. Cardiac: VSD, PDA, tetralogy of Fallot, ASD, right-sided aortic arch
2. Genitourinary: renal agenesis, horseshoe kidney, polycystic kidneys, hypospadias
3. Gastrointestinal: imperforate anus, duodenal atresia, malrotation, Meckel's diverticulum, annular pancreas
4. Musculoskeletal: hemivertebrae, Amelia, poly- and syndactyly, rib malformation, scoliosis

So what are the examination findings in TOF?

It may just be witnessing the historical complaints (above), but a thorough search for all the associated congenital abnormalities must be made

What are the investigations?	**Prenatal**: USS of pregnant uterus may reveal the following:
	1. Polyhydramnios
	2. Absence of a fluid-filled stomach (liquor can't get past atresia)
	3. Small fetal abdomen or fetal size
	4. Distended oesophageal pouch
	Postnatal: a CXR is usually all that is needed. It may show:
	1. Tracheal compression and deviation
	2. Absence of gastric bubble (this indicates oesophageal atresia with a **distal** TOF as tracheal air bypasses atresia)
What is the management?	Surgical repair of the fistula
What are the causes of acquired TOF?	1. Tumour
	2. Infection
	3. Ruptured oesophageal fistulae
	4. Trauma (including iatrogenic during attempted intubation)

DIAPHRAGMATIC HERNIAE

What is a diaphragmatic hernia?	Herniation of abdominal contents through the diaphragm and into the thoracic cavity. It may be congenital or acquired
What types of congenital ones do you know of?	2 main types:
	1. Bochdalek hernia
	2. Morgagni hernia
	Hiatus herniae may also occur congenitally, but are more commonly acquired, occurring in adults
Which one is most common?	Bochdalek herniae (left-sided ones, 90%)
What are their main differences?	See Table 7.1

PART III

Table 7.1

	Bochdalek	Morgagni
Location	Occurs in the posterolateral portions of the diaphragm via the **foramen of Bochdalek** (syn. pleuroperitoneal canal), which occurs at the diaphragmatic dome posteriorly	Occurs anteriorly via the **foramen of Morgagni**, a defect between the sternal and costal attachments of the diaphragm
Side	More common on **left**	More common on the **right**
Contents	**Left**: small and large bowel and solid organs (eg liver) **Right**: liver and a portion of large bowel only **All** herniae tend to have **no sac**	Usually **transverse colon** due to its position
Presentation	Presents in neonates and infants. **Classic triad:** 1. Respiratory distress 2. Apparent dextrocardia 3. Flat 'scaphoid' abdomen	Mainly presents in adults as subacute bowel obstruction, but is usually symptom-free
Investigations	**CXR** may show the following: 1. Abnormally placed stomach (pass NGT to aid in locating it) 2. Loops of bowel in thoracic cavity 3. Cardiac shift 4. Hypoplastic lung on side of herniation or a pneumothorax Perform **echocardiogram**, as up to 25% have associated congenital cardiac defects	
Treatment	Surgical repair, and placement of chest tube if pneumothorax present	

ABDOMEN

HERNIAE AND HYDROCOELES

INGUINAL

What are the important statistics regarding paediatric herniae?

Statistically:
1. M:F = 9:1
2. Indirect:direct = 99:1
3. 5% males are born with an inguinal hernia
4. Side: R>L>bilateral (75:20:5)
5. Hernia repair is the most common paediatric surgery performed

What conditions are associated with an increased risk of inguinal herniae?

1. Prematurity and low birth weight
2. Urological conditions (epispadias, hypospadias, undescended testes)
3. Abdominal wall defects (exomphalos, gastroschisis)

How does it present?

May be difficult to detect clinically. May present as a groin lump which is exaggerated during crying, but disappears at rest

What type of inguinal hernia is most common in children?

Indirect herniae, mainly of the **infantile** type: a **patent processus vaginalis**

What does this mean?

There is a direct communication between the peritoneal cavity and the hernia. (For more on the development of the processus vaginalis, see 'Testes: undescended and ectopic' below)

What is the management?

Surgery is the only treatment: an **inguinal herniotomy** (excision of the hernial sac)

Which cases are considered urgent?

1. Cases in children <1 year old
2. Incarcerated or strangulated herniae

PART III

UMBILICAL AND PARAUMBILICAL

What is the difference between an umbilical and paraumbilical hernia?

An **umbilical hernia** occurs through a weakness in the actual umbilical cicatrix (scar)

A **paraumbilical hernia** occurs through a defect *adjacent* to the cicatrix

Who are more prone to getting these herniae?

Afro-Caribbean populations

What is the usual content?

Both usually contain omentum

What are the treatment options?

Surgical. Either a **mesh repair** or a **Mayo repair** is done. In both, the hernia is reduced and the sac is excised. Then, in the former, a prolene mesh is used to close the defect. In the latter, the cut edges are overlapped ('vest over pants') and sutured together with prolene

What is the rule of 3s in umbilical herniae in infants?

1. Occurs in **3%** of live births
2. Only **3:1000** need repair
3. Repair done only after **age 3**
4. Recur in **3rd trimester** of pregnancy

HYDROCOELE

What is a hydrocoele?

An abnormal collection of fluid in the processus vaginalis

What types do you know of?

Congenital and acquired.
Congenital:
1. **Vaginal**: only the tunica vaginalis part of the processus vaginalis contains fluid (most common)
2. **Infantile**: fluid fills the processus vaginalis up to the external ring
3. **Congenital (as well)**: the entire processus vaginalis is patent with direct communication between the peritoneal cavity and the scrotum (syn. **congenital hernia**; see below)

4. **Hydrocoele of the cord**: only a discrete portion of the processus vaginalis is patent and fluid-filled

Acquired:
1. Primary or idiopathic
2. Secondary to testicular disease (e.g. infection, trauma, carcinoma, TB)

Who gets hydrocoeles?

Mainly middle-aged and elderly men, despite the hydrocoeles being of the congenital variety; children and infants get them as well, however

How does it present?

As a painless scrotal swelling

How is it differentiated from a hernia clinically?

You can get above it (ie you can palpate the spermatic cord above it); it transilluminates; it has no cough impulse. This differs from a hernia which you *cannot* get above, and which *does* have a cough impulse (unless strangulated)

Which hydrocoele is the exception to this rule?

Congenital hydrocoeles with a fully patent processus vaginalis, hence the alternative name of **congenital herniae**

How is the diagnosis made?

History, examination and USS. Aspiration of fluid may also be diagnostic, but should not be done before USS is obtained

What is the treatment?

Surgical excision: the hydrocoele is incised via a trans-scrotal incision, and drained of its fluid. The empty sac is then invaginated on itself and **marsupialised**, thus preventing re-collection of fluid. This is done via either Lord's or Jabolet's approach

PART III

Why not just aspirate them?

Because of high risk of recurrence (though can be done in the interim while the patient is waiting for an operation, if swelling is big enough to cause discomfort)

EXOMPHALOS AND GASTROSCHISIS

What is the basis of exomphalos and gastroschisis?

They are both due to congenital abdominal wall defects

What is an exomphalos?

Herniation of the **mid-gut** through the **umbilical ring** and into the **umbilical cord**, and its failure to return to the **coelom** (fetal abdominal cavity) during early fetal life. (Syn. **omphalocoele**)

What causes this?

Defective mesodermal growth causing failure of central fusion of the umbilical ring

What types of exomphalos are there?

2 types: exomphalos minor and major

What is the difference?

Exomphalos minor: relatively small sac with umbilical cord attached to its summit.
Exomphalos major: very large sac which contains loops of large and small bowel and almost always part of the liver. The umbilical cord is attached to the inferior aspect of the sac

What is gastroschisis?

Herniation of the mid-gut through an abdominal wall defect, usually situated to the right of the umbilicus

Besides location, what is the main difference between them both?

The **covering** of the herniated bowel:
Exomphalos: covered by a **semi-translucent sac** (which may rupture during birth), which comprises the same 3 layers that make up the umbilical cord into which it herniates (outer amniotic membrane, middle Wharton's jelly and inner peritoneum)
Gastroschisis: there is **no cover**; it is a direct herniation through the abdominal wall, not involving the umbilical cord, and so bowel is **directly exposed**

What are the prenatal factors which may indicate these conditions?

Maternal polyhydramnios and raised maternal serum α-fetoprotein (MSAFP)

What is the danger?

Intestinal inflammation, which may occur in gastroschisis or a ruptured omphalocoele

What is the management?

Exomphalos minor: reduce sac contents back into peritoneal cavity by twisting the umbilical cord, and apply strapping for 14 days
Exomphalos major: operation within first few hours of life to replace abdominal contents within the peritoneal cavity before the sac bursts
Gastroschisis: as with exomphalos major, except that the absence of a sac makes it a non-issue. Treating bowel inflammation pre-op facilitates reduction of the bowel

What is the technical difficulty of the operation?

The peritoneal cavity to small to accommodate the bowel contents. Attempting to fit contents all at once may result in respiratory compromise due to splinting of the diaphragm, and compromise of venous return

How is this overcome?	1. By undermining skin flaps and making relaxing incisions in loins to bring defect edges over sac 2. By aspirating bowel contents via an NGT for several days to keep the bowel decompressed
When is the actual abdominal wall defect repaired?	It can be delayed for months to years after the initial operation
What is Beckwith-Wiedemann syndrome?	A triad of the following: 1. Exomphalos 2. Macroglossia (large tongue) 3. Gigantism Affected babies are also prone to developing: 1. Hypoglycaemia (2ry to islet-cell hyperplasia) 2. Visceromegaly 3. Large, rounded facial features
What is prune belly syndrome?	A syndrome of abdominal wall dysplasia. It may consist of the following: 1. Thin, flaccid abdominal wall 2. Bladder hypertrophy with dilation of the renal system 3. Male infertility due to absence of the prostate gland which produces seminal fluid 95% of babies with this syndrome are male

PYLORIC STENOSIS

What is it?	Hypertrophy of the musculature of the pylorus of the stomach of unknown aetiology with stenosis of its lumen
What is the incidence?	4:1000 live births
Who usually gets it?	Usually the first-born male

When do symptoms usually occur?	Between the 3rd and 6th week of life (*key point!!*)
What are the symptoms?	As follows: 1. Vomiting, usually **non-bilious** as the stenosis is **proximal** to the Ampulla of Vater in the 2nd part of the duodenum, into which the biliary tree drains (*another key point!!*) 2. Visible lump, which can be palpated just right of the epigastrium below the liver, especially during feeding. It is an **olive-shaped mass**, and is sometimes known as the **olive sign** 3. Visible peristalsis, especially during feeding 4. Constipation, as minimal fluids pass stenosis, resulting in 'goat-pellet stools' 5. Weight loss
What may prolonged vomiting lead to?	Hypokalaemic, hypochloraemic metabolic alkalosis with a paradoxical aciduria
What are the investigations?	Mainly a clinical diagnosis, but a Ba meal will show the stenosis and elongation of the pylorus
What is the definitive management?	**Ramstedt's operation**: the pyloric musculature is divided down to mucosa without breaching it, causing it to bulge into the pyloric incision, and hence widening the lumen. Make sure electrolyte disturbances have been addressed first

PART III

How can the derivatives of the foregut be remembered?	*Mnemonic:* **L**ive **D**eveloping **E**mbyronic **G**ut **P**roduces **L**iquid **S**tool **L**ungs **D**uodenum (up to ampulla of Vater) o**E**sophagus **G**all bladder **P**ancreas **L**iver **S**tomach

BOWEL ATRESIA

DUODENAL ATRESIA

What is it?	Congenital atresia of the lumen of the duodenum
Which part of the duodenum is usually affected?	The 2nd part of the duodenum, around the Ampulla of Vater, the drainage point of bile from the biliary tree
What is the Ampulla of Vater the anatomical landmark for?	It marks the junction of the foregut and the midgut
How does duodenal atresia present?	With vomiting **from birth**, the vomitus is usually **bilious**. (*Key points!* Compare with pyloric stenosis above). There is rapid weight loss as a result
What are the investigations?	**Prenatal**: maternal abdominal USS may reveal polyhydramnios and a fetal distended, fluid-filled stomach (fluid cannot pass atretic portion). There may also be other congenital abnormalities (eg cardiac) **Post-natally**: erect and supine AXR will reveal a **double-bubble sign** (gas bubble in stomach proximal to a gas bubble in proximal part of duodenum). The rest of the bowel will be gas-free, suggesting atresia which swallowed air cannot by-pass

What is the definitive management?

A **duodenoduodenostomy** (the lumen of the duodenum proximal and distal to the atretic segment are anastomosed, hence by-passing the atretic segment), or a **duodenojejunostomy** (higher post-op complications)

ANORECTAL AGENESIS

What is this?

A spectrum of congenital anomalies occurring secondary to interference with anorectal structural development

How common are these?

Relatively common, minor defects occurring in 1:500 live births, major defects occurring in 1:5000

Do the anal canal and rectum develop as one?

Yes. They develop from the dorsal portion of the hindgut or **cloacal cavity**. This dorsal portion is separated from the ventrally situated urethra and bladder by the **urorectal septum** in the midline

What about the anus itself?

This develops as a fusion of the **anal tubercles** and an external invagination known as the **proctodeum**. This invaginates toward the anorectal canal, and is separated from it by the **anal membrane**. This membrane breaks down by the 8th week of gestation

What range of anomalies can occur?

Anomalies are separated into **high** and **low** ones depending on their relation to the **levator ani muscle complex**. Examples are:
1. Anal stenosis (low)
2. Imperforate anus (incomplete breakdown of anal membrane; low)
3. Anal agenesis (low)

PART III

4. Complete failure of rectal descent and invagination of proctodeum (high)

What are these anomalies frequently associated with?

Fistulae, the type depending on whether they are high or low, and whether the child is male or female. Examples are:
1. Recto-urethral
2. Rectovaginal
3. Rectoprostatic

What is the typical history?

A newborn infant who fails to pass meconium within the 1st 24 hours of life
Less severe cases may occur with gradual constipation and abdominal distension

What are the examination findings?

In either sex: a flat perineum with a short sacrum suggests a high lesion
In females: a single perineal opening suggests an anomaly present (there should be 2: a vaginal and an anal opening)
In males: look for signs of recto-urethral or rectoprostatic fistulae (meconium at penile meatus or in urine, or pneumaturia)

What are the investigations?

AXR usually cinches the diagnosis. Film done with baby in kneeling position. A coin (or other radio-opaque marker) is placed on the perineum as a marker

What is the management?

Surgery, tailored to the type of anomaly present.
Generally, in high lesions, a colostomy is fashioned in the first instance until definitive repair can occur at a later date

MECKEL'S DIVERTICULUM

What is Meckel's diverticulum?

A true diverticulum occurring on the **antimesenteric** border of the terminal ileum. It represents the embryological remnant of the **vitello-intestinal** duct, and has the following properties:
- Occurs in **2%** of the population
- Has a **2:1** male:female ratio
- Is approximately **2 inches** long
- Is found **2 feet** from the ileocaecal junction
- **1 in 2** will contain ectopic tissue (gastric of pancreatic)
- Only **2%** are symptomatic
- Important cause of rectal bleeding in **under 2s**

This is the **rule of 2s**

Why does it present like an appendicitis?

If ectopic gastric mucosa present, may ulcerate and/or perforate

How is it diagnosed?

Incidentally at operation or clinically if symptomatic. Can be scanned using IV **technetium pertechnetate** (Meckel's scan), which is preferentially taken up by gastric mucosa

How is it treated?

Surgical excision

INTUSSUSCEPTION

What is it?

The telescoping, prolapse or invagination of one segment of bowel (**intussusceptum**) in an immediately adjacent one (**intussuscipiens**), usually a proximal segment into a distal one

Which type of intussusception is most common?

Ileocolic (terminal ileum into proximal colon)

Why?

Thought to be due to a high aggregation of **Peyer's patches** (lymphoid aggregates) in the terminal ileal wall which 'drag' the ileum into the colon, especially when swollen during inflammation

What are the other causes?

1. Protrusion of masses into lumen of bowel
   a. Polyp (esp. in Peutz–Jeghers syndrome where intussusception may be recurrent)
   b. Submucous lipoma
   c. Papilliferous carcinoma
2. Meckel's diverticulum
3. Cystic fibrosis
4. Change in diet
5. Idiopathic (most common; 90%)

Who gets it?

Usually male infants (M:F = 3:1) between the ages of 3 to 12 months

What is the big risk with intussusception?

Early bowel gangrene as the blood supply of the inner layers of the intussusception may be compromised, especially in a tight invagination

How does it present?

Classically with the following triad:
1. Colicky abdominal pain lasting for 10–20 min
2. Vomiting
3. Red-currant jelly stool (blood and mucus mix *per rectum*)

The colicky abdominal pain, which coincides with a bout of intussusception, usually punctuates long spells of the child seemingly being absolutely fine

What are the examination findings?	There may be nothing to palpate on the abdomen, but during intussusception, there may be a firm **sausage-shaped mass** palpable in the RUQ. Rectal exam may reveal the classic **red-currant jelly stool**
What is the investigation of choice?	A **barium enema**. This will cinch the diagnosis, *and* may reduce the intussusception via a hydrostatic pressure (it will push the intussusceptum out of the intussuscipiens)
What is the management?	**Conservative**: barium enema (high success rate) **Surgical**: operative reduction

HIRSCHSPRUNG'S DISEASE

What is it?	An arrest in the migration of ganglionic cells within the colon and rectum leading to an absence of parasympathetic ganglion cells in the **myenteric** and **submucosal plexus** of the rectum and/or colon
What is the result?	An aganglionic segment of large bowel
Who gets it?	Males (M:F = 4:1), during the 1st 2 years of life
Does it run in families?	Yes, in about 30% of cases
What is Hirschsprung's disease strongly associated with?	Downs' syndrome
How does it present?	**Newborns** may present with gross abdominal distension, vomiting and failure to pass meconium within the first 48 hours of life

Older children may present with **chronic constipation**, but *without* faecal soiling due to overflow incontinence seen in constipation of other causes

Nearly all kids are malnourished

What are the examination findings?

A malnourished child with a grossly distended abdomen with tympany and signs of large bowel obstruction. Rectal exam usually reveals an **empty rectum** (in contrast to other causes of constipation)

What are the investigations?

AXR will show faecal impaction with distended loops of proximal bowel and no gas in the rectum

Rectal manometry shows failure of rectum to relax on balloon inflation

Rectal biopsy reveals aganglionic segment

What is the management?

Medical: as for any case of bowel obstruction: 'drip and suck' regime (IV fluids and NGT; keep child NBM). Attempt enemas

Surgical: colostomy proximal to aganglionic segment and resection of segment, followed by pull-through procedure of proximal normal segment as a staged procedure at a later date

What is Hirschsprung's enterocolitis?

A potentially fatal outcome of the disease presenting with fever, malaise, vomiting and foul-smelling, often bloody diarrhoea. Gut necrosis and perforation may ensue

NECROTISING ENTEROCOLITIS (NEC)

What is it?	An acute inflammatory disease occurring in the intestines of premature and under-weight newborn infants; necrosis of intestinal tissue may follow, with severe systemic effects
What is its incidence?	0.5–1:1000 live births
What are the causes?	Unknown, but bacterial infection and hypoxia are postulated. It is known to sometimes follow umbilical artery catheterisation
How does it present?	With the following: 1. Feeding problems 2. Abdominal distension 3. Bright red blood *per rectum* (late) 4. Apnoeic spells 5. Lethargy
And on examination?	Can be divided into abdominal and systemic: **Abdominal**: distended abdomen, tender on palpation or peritonitic, with ↓ bowel sounds (ileus). A **mass** may be palpable. The abdominal wall may be erythematous (late sign). There may be bright red blood PR **Systemic**: fever and tachycardia; in the late stages, the child may show signs of septic shock with ↓ peripheral perfusion and cardiovascular collapse (**fulminant NEC**). A DIC may ensue and present as a **bleeding diathesis**
What are the investigations?	**Blood investigations**: 1. FBC: ↓platelets, ↑WBC with left shift (neutrophilia)

PART III

1. U&E: ↓Na or other metabolic derangements
2. ABG: metabolic acidosis
3. Clotting: DIC picture (↑PT, ↑aPTT, ↓fibrinogen, ↑FDP)

Radiology: AXR will show:

1. Distended bowel loops
2. Intramural gas (gas within the bowel wall; syn. **pneumatosis intestinalis**: *pathognomonic* for NEC!)
3. Free abdominal air (suggests bowel perforation)
4. Portal venous gas (seen as line shadows over liver and represents air in portal system, a grave sign)

What is the management?

Medical first!

1. Resuscitate, resuscitate, resuscitate:
   a. IV fluids
   b. NBM/NGT
   c. Catheterise and monitor I/O
2. IV broad spectrum antibiotics for 7–14 days depending on severity
3. Consider PICU for inotropic support if shocked

When is surgery indicated?

1. If there is ↑ peritonitis
2. If there is evidence of perforated bowel (peritonitis, free abdominal gas on X-ray)
3. If medical management fails
4. If there is an abdominal mass present

What surgery is performed?

Either of the following:

1. Resection of affected segment and fashioning of an ileostomy with mucous fistula, with re-anastomosis done at a later stage
2. Resection of affected segment with primary anastomosis

What is the prognosis of NEC?

Poor overall: 20% mortality in those requiring only medical treatment; 30% in those progressing to surgery

What is thought to protect against NEC?

Breast-feeding

VOLVULUS NEONATORUM

What is it?

Volvulus (twisting on itself) of the **midgut** in the newborn, resulting in intestinal obstruction

What predisposes to it?

Arrested rotation: the gut rotates only 90° instead of its normal counter clockwise 270° before returning to the abdominal cavity during fetal development. This means that the colon and caecum are the first to return from the umbilical cord to the abdomen and settle in the LUQ, with later returning loops lying more and more to the right

So how does this arrested rotation cause volvulus neonatorum?

The abnormally placed caecum and the small intestine attached to it float freely on a narrow mesenteric pedicle and are therefore free to twist

How does the infant present?

With symptoms of mechanical intestinal obstruction: distended abdomen, colicky abdominal pain, vomiting and obstipation

What are the radiological findings?

AXR will show abnormally placed bowel in keeping with arrested rotation, together with distended loops of bowel

What is the management?

'Drip and suck' regime (NBM, NGT, IV fluids), and laparotomy with untwisting of the volvulus (untwist in a clockwise fashion)

PART III

What else does arrested rotation predispose to?	The formation of abnormal peritoneal bands, in particular a transduodenal band running from the caecum to the right side of the abdomen across the 2nd part of the duodenum. The presentation is almost identical to that of duodenal atresia (see before)
What is this transduodenal band also called?	A **Ladd band**

HEPATOBILIARY AND PANCREATIC CONDITIONS

BILIARY ATRESIA

What is it?	A discontinuity in the patency of the biliary tree resulting in obstruction of bile flow and subsequent **cholestatic jaundice**
What types do you know of?	Two main types: **postnatal** and **fetal**. **Postnatal**: more common (65–90%); comprises an isolated atresia of the biliary tree **Fetal**: atresia is associated with situs inversus or poly-/asplenia ± other congenital abnormalities
What are the causes?	**Fetal atresia**: thought to be due to a failure in embryogenesis **Postnatal atresia**: infection (possibly viral, ?CMV) has been postulated
What types of postnatal atresias are there?	Again, 2 main types: **correctable** and **non-correctable**. Correctable atresias are those in which there is at least *some* communication with the intrahepatic bile ducts. In non-correctable cases, no such communication exists (see Figure 7.2)

Figure 7.2

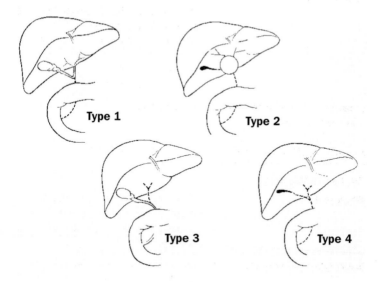

Type 1

Type 2

Type 3

Type 4

What are the clinical features?

1. Obstructive jaundice by the 2nd week of life
2. Dark urine and pale stools
3. Pruritis (dermal bile salt collection)
4. Skin xanthomas (hypercholesterolaemia)
5. Clubbing

How is it diagnosed?

Blood investigations: show an obstructive jaundice type picture ($\uparrow$bilirubin, $\uparrow\uparrow$ALP, $\uparrow$AST)

Radiology:

1. **USS**: shows defect and to r/o other differentials
2. **Radioisotope scanning**: failure of tree to be visualised and the isotope to reach intestine via biliary tree suggests diagnosis

What is the treatment?

Correctable cases: anastomosis of a jejunal loop to the patent portion of the biliary tree in communication with the intrahepatic ducts

'Non-correctable' cases: anastomosis of a jejunal loop directly to the intrahepatic ducts by attaching it flush with the liver surface at the porta hepatis (**portojejunostomy** or **Kasai procedure**)

What is the overall prognosis of biliary atresia?

Poor

CHOLEDOCHAL CYST

What is it?

An out-pouching of the wall of the biliary tree due to a weakness of part or all of its wall

What is the most common type?

Fusiform dilation: the entire wall of a particular segment is weak, causing a symmetrical dilation (see Figure 7.3)

Figure 7.3

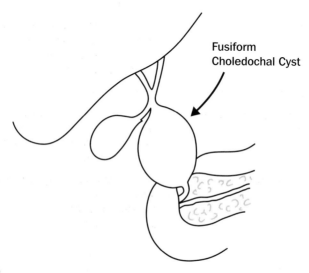

Fusiform
Choledochal Cyst

Who gets it?	Females (F:M = 4:1); more common in Japanese
How does it present?	Symptoms appear at age 6 months and older: 1. Intermittent obstructive jaundice 2. Upper abdominal pain 3. Pyrexia (if infection present) 4. Abdominal mass (cyst can contain up to 2 l)
What are the risks of these cysts?	Eventual **biliary cirrhosis** or **chemical peritonitis** 2ry to cyst rupture, with possible death. Cysts prone to development of **carcinoma**
How are they diagnosed?	USS
What is the treatment?	Excision of cyst and choledochojejunostomy (anastomosis of biliary tree to jejunum)

ANNULAR PANCREAS

What is it?	A ring of pancreatic tissue surrounding the 2nd or 3rd part of the duodenum, and hence predisposing to obstructive vomiting
How does it occur?	Failure of the ventral pancreatic bud to completely rotate (pancreas develops from a ventral and dorsal bud which rotate and fuse)
What is it associated with?	High incidence in Down's syndrome
What is the nature of the vomitus?	Depends on whether the annular pancreas occurs proximal or distal to the Ampulla of Vater (non-bilious or bilious respectively)
What is the treatment?	Bypass of the constricting pancreatic tissue either by duodenoduodenostomy or duodenojejunostomy

PART III

131

GENITO-URINARY

APPLIED ANATOMY

What are the stages of testicular descent?

2nd month: intra-abdominal structure
End of 4th month: testis at deep inguinal ring
7th month: within inguinal canal
Shortly after birth: within scrotum

What precedes the testis during descent?

The gubernaculum

What is the gubernaculum?

A mesenchymal condensation attached to the inferior pole of the testis, whose gradual contraction is thought to drag the testis behind it into the scrotum where it eventually attaches

What does the testis descend in?

A peritoneal invagination, the **processus vaginalis**

What is the fate of the processus vaginalis?

Its lumen obliterates shortly after birth, leaving only a small portion surrounding the testis, the **tunica vaginalis**, attached to its posterior and lateral surfaces

What is the penis made up of?

Two **corpora cavernosa** (sing. corpus cavernosum), the erectile portions of the penis which abut the glans penis. The **glans penis** is the dilated end part of the **corpus spongiosum**, which contains the penile urethra

What type of epithelium is the penile urethra made up of?

Transitional cell epithelium for most of its length, except for its distal portion which is squamous

ANOMALIES OF THE KIDNEY AND URETER

What is Potter syndrome?

Potter syndrome, which causes a typical physical appearance, is the result of oligohydramnios secondary to renal diseases such as bilateral renal agenesis. Other causes of Potter syndrome include obstructive uropathy, autosomal recessive polycystic kidney disease, and renal hypoplasia.

How can the features of Potter syndrome be remembered?

Mnemonic: **POTTER**
Pulmonary hypoplasia
Oligohydramnios (↓ liquor volume)
Twisted skin (wrinkled skin)
Twisted face (Potter facies)
Extremity defects
Renal agenesis (bilateral)

HORSESHOE KIDNEY

What is it?

A developmental abnormality of the kidney in which the kidney is, as the name implies, one entire **horseshoed mass**, fused at the lower poles, and lying in an abnormal position. (Very rarely, the *upper* poles are fused)

What position is this?

The fused lower poles are usually at the level of L4

Why is this?

Because the fused lower poles hook around the inferior mesenteric artery of the abdominal aorta, which prevents further upward migration during the kidneys' fetal ascent

Are the adrenal glands also affected?

No. They develop separately from the kidneys (neural crest origin) and are found in their normal positions

What is the incidence?

About 1:1000 found at autopsy

PART III

What is its significance?

The fashion in which the ureters enter each kidney is more angulated, making urinary stasis more likely to occur, and hence predisposing to UTI (including TB) and calculi

How does it present?

Oftentimes it is an incidental finding either during radiology for other causes, or at autopsy. In the very young, it may present as a suprapubic mass. Otherwise, it may be the cause of repeated UTI's/calculi

How is it diagnosed?

Either by KUB USS or IVU

What is the management?

No intervention necessary. Division of the lower poles only done for access to other structures, as during abdominal aortic aneurysm repair

POLYCYSTIC KIDNEY

What is it?

Hereditary, cystic, gross enlargement of the kidneys

What type of inheritance is it?

Autosomal dominant

What are the clinical features?

These usually occur in adulthood:
1. Renal enlargement
2. Flank pain (dragging sensation)
3. Pyelonephritis (most common complication)
4. Haematuria
5. Hypertension
6. Renal failure

How is it diagnosed?

KUB USS and IVU

PHIMOSIS, PARAPHIMOSIS AND CIRCUMCISION

What are the indications for circumcision?

1. Religious or cultural reasons (most common)
2. Phimosis/paraphimosis (see below)
3. Recurrent balanitis (infection under prepuce)
4. Torn or tight frenulum

What is phimosis?

The inability to retract the distal prepuce (foreskin) over the glans penis

What types of phimosis are there?

Congenital (physiological) and acquired:

Congenital (physiological): adhesions exist between the prepuce and the glans penis. These adhesions usually resolve by themselves (sometimes by the time the child is a teenager). It does not cause problems such as obstruction

Acquired: usually due to recurrent balanitis; poor hygiene is a contributing factor

How can you tell the difference clinically?

In congenital phimosis, the foreskin 'pouts', whereas it does not in acquired phimosis (see Figure 7.4)

PART III

Figure 7.4

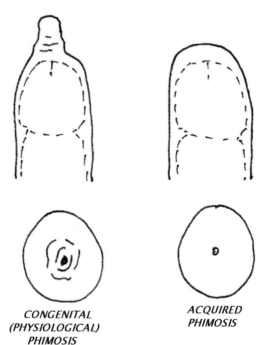

CONGENITAL
(PHYSIOLOGICAL)
PHIMOSIS

ACQUIRED
PHIMOSIS

What is paraphimosis?

Entrapment of the retracted prepuce behind the coronal sulcus. Causes oedema of the penile head, aggravating the condition. This condition is painful and is a **urological emergency**

How is paraphimosis managed?

By firmly squeezing the penile head to empty it of its oedema (anaesthetise the penis first by performing a lignocaine ring block *without* adrenaline), so facilitating reduction of the prepuce. Aspiration of oedema with a large needle (16 G) may be necessary. If all else fails, perform a dorsal slit in the foreskin to release it

HYPOSPADIAS, EPISPADIAS AND BLADDER EXSTROPHY

HYPOSPADIAS

What is hypospadias?

An abnormality of anterior urethral development in which the urethral opening is ectopically located on the **ventrum** (underside) of the penis proximal to the tip of the glans penis. The opening may be as proximal as the scrotum or perineum (see Figure 7.5)

Figure 7.5

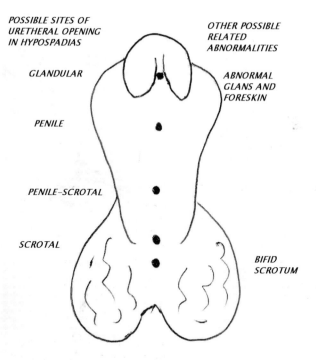

POSSIBLE SITES OF URETHERAL OPENING IN HYPOSPADIAS

OTHER POSSIBLE RELATED ABNORMALITIES

GLANDULAR

ABNORMAL GLANS AND FORESKIN

PENILE

PENILE–SCROTAL

SCROTAL

BIFID SCROTUM

What is the actual developmental pathology?	Failure of complete fusion of the genital folds and glandular urethra. Genetic and endocrine factors have been postulated
What is its incidence?	1:500 live birth male infants. More common in Jewish races
What often accompanies hypospadias?	A curvature in the penis known as a **chordee**. There may also be an abnormal foreskin
How does it present?	Usually discovered at birth
What are the clinical findings?	Chordee, a ventrally incomplete foreskin, and a ventrally placed urethral opening anywhere from proximal to the glans to the scrotum If the urethral opening is scrotal, a **bifid scrotum** (2 separate hemi-scrotums) may also be found Look out for ectopic testes or cryptorchidism (see below) and inguinal herniae, which may co-exist
What is the management?	Surgical repair at age 6–18 months: 1. Urethroplasty: create a normal urethra which opens via a meatus at the penile tip 2. Glansplasty: create a normal, conical glans 3. Orthoplasty: straighten any chordee present These will ensure that the child will be able to: 1. Urinate normally instead of having to sit down 2. Have normal future sexual intercourse
What are the risks of hypospadias surgery?	Urethral fistula and stricture
What is forbidden in a child with hypospadias?	Circumcision! The foreskin is used during urethroplasty

EPISPADIAS AND BLADDER EXSTROPHY

What is epispadias?

An abnormality of anterior urethral development in which the urethral opening is ectopically located on the **dorsum** (topside) of the penis proximal to the tip of the glans penis. Genital abnormalities may be associated

Do only boys get it?

No. Unlike hypospadias, girls may have epispadias as well, with **clitoral** abnormalities. It is much more uncommon in girls, however, and associated with more abnormalities

What is bladder exstrophy?

A congenital abnormality in which the bladder is exposed, inside out, and protrudes through the abdominal wall

Do these two conditions occur together?

They can. The **exstrophy–epispadias complex** comprises a spectrum of congenital abnormalities that includes classic bladder exstrophy, epispadias, cloacal exstrophy, and several variants

How common are they?

Rare!

Bladder exstrophy:	3:100,000 live births
Epispadias (male):	1:117,000 live births
Epispadias (female):	1:484,000 live births

What is the basis of the complex?

Instability of the **cloacal membrane** (the cloaca is also known as the **urogenital sinus**, from which urinary and genital organs originate), resulting in its premature rupture before full caudal descent. The outcome is a range of infra-umbilical abnormalities, including genital and urinary tract malformations and anterior abdominal wall defects

What are the clinical findings?	**Boys**: short, broad penis with dorsal slit. Bilateral inguinal herniae and cryptorchidism may be present **Girls**: a cleft clitoris **Both sexes**: the deep red mucous membrane of the posterior bladder wall protrudes through an abdominal wall defect and readily bleeds
Radiology?	Plain films may show separation of the pubis, which may occur in both sexes
How is it managed?	**Surgical repair** is performed within the 1st 48 hours of birth. It involves: 1. Separation of the exposed bladder from the abdominal wall bladder repair 2. Repair of the bladder neck and epispadias A catheter is left in to drain the urine from the bladder through the abdominal wall. A second catheter is left in the urethra to promote healing
What about the pelvic bones?	If separated, they should be surgically attached to each other. Post-op lower body cast or sling is applied to promote healing. This surgery may be done with the first surgery, or it may be delayed for weeks or months

TESTES: *UNDESCENDED AND ECTOPIC*

APPLIED ANATOMY

What are the stages of testicular descent?	**2nd month**: intra-abdominal structure **End of 4th month**: testis at deep inguinal ring **7th month**: within inguinal canal **Shortly after birth**: within scrotum
What precedes the testis during descent?	The gubernaculum

What is the gubernaculum?	A mesenchymal condensation attached to the inferior pole of the testis, whose gradual contraction is thought to drag the testis behind it into the scrotum where it eventually attaches
What does the testis descend in?	A peritoneal invagination, the **processus vaginalis**
What is the fate of the processus vaginalis?	Its lumen obliterates shortly after birth, leaving only an small portion surrounding the testis, the **tunica vaginalis**, attached to its posterior and lateral surfaces

CLINICAL CONSIDERATIONS

What is the condition of undescended testes also called?	Cryptorchidism
And what *is* cryptorchidism?	The failure of the testis to descend from its intra-abdominal position into the scrotum
What causes it?	Unknown
Can it occur in both testes?	Yes, in ⅓ of patients
In which population does it have a higher incidence?	Premature infants
At what age does the patient present?	At any age, from infancy to adolescence. Most often, parents bring the child in, claiming that they cannot feel the testis
What are the examination findings?	An empty hemiscrotum (or whole scrotum in ⅓ of patients). The testis may be palpated anywhere along its course of descent:

Inguinal canal (most common)   70%
Prescrotal (at external ring)   20%
Abdominal (not palpable)   10%
(see Figure 7.6)

Figure 7.6

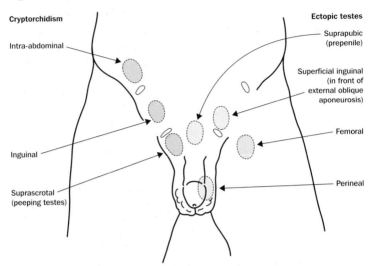

Cryptorchidism

Intra-abdominal

Inguinal

Suprascrotal
(peeping testes)

Ectopic testes

Suprapubic
(prepenile)

Superficial inguinal
(in front of
external oblique
aponeurosis)

Femoral

Perineal

What is important during examination of a child with possible cryptorchidism?

Ensure the child is warm, as he may not have cryptorchidism, but **retractile testes**. In this normal condition of pre-pubertal boys, the **dartos muscle** of the scrotum has a strong reflex, and contracts vigorously (especially in cold environments), causing the testes to retract to the point of being impalpable. They may be coaxed down by warming the child (in a warm bath if necessary) *Attempt milking the testis down*, starting at the deep inguinal ring, along the canal, down to the scrotum (used lubricated finger if necessary)

What should you also examine?

Once retractile testes have been ruled out, examine the areas where an **ectopic testis** may occur. Also examine the penis, as **hypospadias** can sometimes occur as an associated condition (see before).

Other occasional findings are omphalocoele and gastroschisis

What is an ectopic testis?

One which has descended as normal, but to an abnormal location. The likely places include (in descending order):
1. Superficial inguinal pouch (in front of external oblique aponeurosis)
2. Perineum (at root of penis)
3. Suprapubis
4. Femoral region

(see Figure 7.6)

What are the investigations?

USS is the test of choice to confirm cryptorchidism.
CT/MRI are used if USS fails to locate testis. If all imaging fails, a laparoscopic search is performed

What is the management?

Retractile testes: reassurance, as it disappears in adolescence
Cryptorchidism: orchiopexy (fixing of the testis in the scrotum) at age 2–10
Ectopic testis: orchiopexy at age 2–10

What are the risks of cryptorchidism?

1. There is an increased risk of injury in an abnormally placed testis
2. There is also a 20–48 times risk of **malignant change** in the undescended testis (*the undescended testis is also at risk*)

Does this malignant risk decrease with orchiopexy?

No. Follow-up is and education in self-exam is important

What about ectopic testes?

They have the same risks as cryptorchidism.

POSTERIOR URETHRAL VALVES

What are they?

Valves occurring in the posterior urethra, usually below the level of the verumontanum (mound in the prostatic urethra into which drain the seminal vesicles), which may lead to urinary obstruction.
They are usually symmetrical and complete

How do they present?

As **acute urinary obstruction** in the infant. There is a painful suprapubic mass palpable (the distended bladder)
Rarely, if incomplete, they may present in adolescence as chronic urinary obstruction

How can it be diagnosed?

Micturating cystography (dye injected into blood stream, and films taken during micturition after bladder is full): a **dilated urethra** proximal to the valves is seen, and possibly **bladder diverticula** from back-pressure

What is the management?

Trans-urethral valvulotomy

CHAPTER 8: OTOLARYNGOLOGY, HEAD & NECK SURGERY

EAR

APPLIED ANATOMY

Figure 8.1

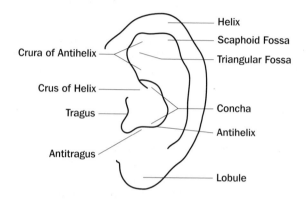

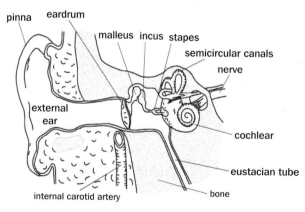

CROSS SECTION OF THE EAR

GENERAL CONCEPTS

How is the ear subdivided?

External ear: pinna (auricle), external meatus, tympanic membrane (TM or eardrum)
Middle ear: ossicles (malleus, incus and stapes), mastoid antrum and air cells, Eustachian tube, facial nerve
Inner ear: cochlea, vestibule, semicircular canals

What are the functions of these?

External ear channels sound towards the eardrum and protects deeper structures
Middle ear is an air-filled cavity, acting as an impedance matching device. Helps transmit sound waves between the environment (air) via the tympanic membrane and ossicles to the oval window of the cochlea (fluid)
Inner ear contains the hearing organ (cochlea), and central balance systems (vestibule and semicircular canals). These are connected to the auditory cortex and cerebellum by the vestibulocochlear nerve.

What should you ask about in the history?

Ear symptoms: the Ds
Deafness (*hearing loss*)
Discomfort (*otalgia*, ear pain)
Discharge (*otorrhoea* – fluid, pus or blood)
Droning (tinnitus)
Dizziness or loss of balance

Associated details: the Ns
Nose (obstruction, discharge)
Nodes (cervical lymphadenopathy)
Natural history of symptoms (onset, progress, etc)
Noise (work or recreational exposure)
Noxious insults (surgery, trauma, ototoxic drugs)
Natal history (family, antenatal, birth, childhood)

How do you examine the ear?

Introduction: ask permission and which ear is better
General inspection of the patient (age, syndromes); look at the external ears first
Otoscopy: start with the better ear, **ask if it is sore**. Use the otoscope (auriscope) *with care.*
Hold it like a pencil, in the same hand as the side of the ear being examined. Rest your little finger on the patient's face. Retract the pinna *gently* with the opposite hand. Gently insert the speculum into the canal and **look**

What should you look for?

Pinna: malformations, scars, infection, trauma
Canal: wax, discharge, oedema, obstruction
TM: landmarks, colour, vascularity and mobility – ask the patient to try the Valsalva manoeuvre

Figure 8.2 Structure of the normal left inner ear

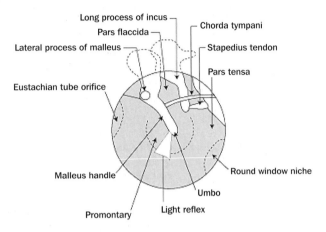

- Long process of incus
- Chorda tympani
- Pars flaccida
- Lateral process of malleus
- Stapedius tendon
- Pars tensa
- Eustachian tube orifice
- Round window niche
- Malleus handle
- Umbo
- Promontary
- Light reflex

| **What else should you examine?** | **Nose**: remember that the Eustachian tube opens at the back of the nose (postnasal space or PNS). A full ear examination *must* exclude pathology here: this usually requires a fine nasal endoscope |
| | **Nodes**: check the draining lymph node groups |

HEARING LOSS (DEAFNESS)

| **How do you classify deafness?** | **Conductive** vs **Sensorineural** **Congenital** vs **Acquired** So take a full **history** and remember the **anatomy** |
| **What are common causes?** | See Table 8.1 |

Table 8.1

Onset	Conductive	Sensorineural
Congenital	Malformations of the external and middle ear + ossicles (rare)	Genetic (family history, syndromes) Antenatal infections, eg Rubella
Acquired	**Wax** **Glue ear** Foreign body Infection Trauma Perforation	**Age related (presbyacusis)** **Noise exposure** Infections (local, perinatal or systemic, eg meningitis) Trauma Vascular events Neoplasia (rare)

What is wax?

Wax is a mixture of secretions (from ceruminous glands of the outer ⅓ of the ear canal), desquamated skin and hair. It is **normal** and **protective**

What is glue ear?

Also known as *otitis media with effusion* (OME), this is a build up of fluid in the middle ear. This reduces TM mobility and produces conductive deafness

Who is affected?

It is commonest in young children, reducing with age. Certain syndromes (eg Down's) predispose to it

What causes glue ear?

Eustachian tube dysfunction, which is seen most often in children, where the tube is short and narrow, and may be blocked at the PNS by big adenoids. In adults, always exclude PNS pathology, eg carcinoma

How does it present?

History: Most commonly speech delay or inattention at home or school – *get the history from the parents*
O/E: TM may be retracted ± middle ear fluid

How is it treated?

Conservatively: watch and wait, it often resolves (approx 3/12)
Surgically: insertion of grommets into the TMs, tubes which help *ventilate* (NOT *drain*) the middle ear, and improve conduction of sound

What is presbyacusis?

This is degenerative, age-related deafness, due to loss of hair cells in the cochlea

What are its characteristics?

Both ears are affected. High frequencies are involved first, so consonants such as 'p' and 't' are not heard well, and the person struggles to *discriminate* between words and different voices in a noisy environment

How is it treated?

Exclude reversible causes first, such as drugs (eg frusemide). **Aids to hearing** are often useful

What types of aids to hearing are available?

Electronic aids:
Behind the ear
In the ear
In the canal
Bone conducting/anchored
Body worn
Cochlear implants
Environmental aids: eg doorbell with flashing lights
Lip reading/signing
Organisations for the deaf, eg Royal National Institute for the Deaf (RNID)

HEARING TESTS

What tests can you perform?

Free field hearing tests check the patient's ability to hear your voice (whispered, normal or loud) at 60 cm, 30 cm and 10 cm. Try random numbers, and mask the hearing of the opposite ear by rubbing the tragus

Tuning fork tests distinguish between **conductive** (external and/or middle ear) and **sensorineural** (inner ear) hearing loss:

Rinne test compares air conduction (AC, when the vibrating tuning fork is held near the ear canal) with bone conduction (BC, when the fork is pressed against the mastoid process). Normally **AC>BC**, called **Rinne positive**. With a conductive loss, **AC<BC**: **Rinne negative**

The **Weber Test** is more sensitive, but *must be used in the context of a Rinne test*. When a vibrating tuning fork is pressed onto the forehead or vertex, the sound is normally heard equally in both ears. If the sound *lateralises* to one ear, this indicates a conductive hearing loss in that ear *or* a sensorineural loss in the *opposite* ear. The results of the Rinne test will show which is which

What other tests are available?

Pure tone audiometry (PTA) is the standard method of recording hearing levels. Sounds are presented to each ear separately using headphones, and the patient presses a button each time a sound is heard. Hearing thresholds (in decibels, dB) for standard frequencies (Hz) are plotted on a graph. AC and BC can be compared for each ear. Needs compliance, so not useful for young children

Figure 8.3

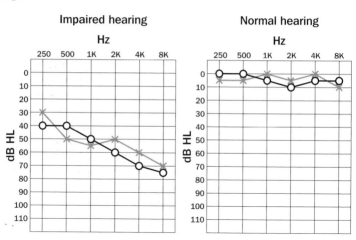

Impaired hearing   Normal hearing

O Right ear
× Left ear

Impedance tympanometry

assesses the mobility of the TM and can show Eustachian tube dysfunction and middle ear fluid (as in glue ear). A probe in the canal emits tones which bounce off the TM, and a microphone picks these up. A flat graph suggests glue ear or a TM perforation. Useful for any age of patient

Figure 8.4

TYMPANOGRAMS

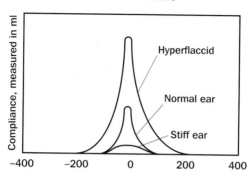

Pressure at which peak compliance occurs,
measured in decapascals

What extra hearing tests are used for young children?	**Otoacoustic emission tests** are useful for screening neonates: acoustic stimulation of the normal cochlea produces low-level sound, detected by a microphone
	Distraction testing involves trying to elicit a head-turning response when sounds are presented to a child (who is *distracted* by playing with an assistant)
	Brainstem-evoked response audiometry measures the brain's responses to sound. The child must be asleep or anaesthetised.

EAR PAIN (OTALGIA)

How is otalgia classified?

> **Remember to classify answers in *simple* terms**
> eg anatomical, local vs general, direct vs indirect, acute vs chronic, and common *then* rare

Otalgia can arise from the **ear** itself (**otologic otalgia**) or can be referred from **elsewhere** (**non-otologic otalgia**)

What are the main *otologic* causes?

Infections of the pinna (cellulitis/ perichondritis) the ear canal (otitis externa) the TM (myringitis) the middle ear (acute otitis media) the mastoid (acute mastoiditis)
Trauma: **direct** (eg with a cotton bud or stick); **indirect** (eg barotrauma from diving)
Neoplasia: eg SCC in the ear canal (rare)

OTITIS EXTERNA

What is otitis externa (OE)?

Infection of the ear canal. It is *common*

Who is affected?

Adults are more often affected. Risk factors include **local insults** (eg swimming in dirty water, trauma with cotton buds or syringing) and **general problems** (eg diabetes and skin disorders)

What organisms cause it?

Bacteria: *Pseudomonas,* Streptococci, Staphylococci
Fungi: *Aspergillus, Candida*

What are the symptoms?

Irritation and pruritus, then pain and creamy, smelly discharge

What are the signs?

Both ears are often involved. Pain may be severe, so insert the otoscope gently. The canal wall may be oedematous, narrowing the lumen, and discharge often obstructs views to the TM.
Systemic upset is unusual

How is OE treated?	**Prevention**: avoid/treat the risk factors above **Aural toilet**: microsuction of the discharge under the microscope in ENT clinic + swab for M/C/S **Ear drops**: according to the causative agent, eg gentamicin, gramicidin, ciprofloxacin **Analgesia**: paracetamol, codeine, NSAIDs
What complication can occur?	**Malignant otitis externa**: a chronic, aggressive form of OE. This is a **misnomer** as it is *not* a cancer, but rather a form of **osteomyelitis of the temporal bone** causing invasive destruction into the middle ear, nerves and brain. Caused by *Pseudomonas* in (elderly) **diabetics**. May be hard to distinguish from SCC

ACUTE OTITIS MEDIA

What is acute otitis media?	Inflammation of the middle ear, usually following URTI, where organisms ascend via the Eustachian tube. This is *not* glue ear
Who is affected?	Very common in young children, rare in adults
What organisms cause it?	**Bacteria**: *Pneumococcus, Haemophilus influenzae, Moraxella catarrhalis*
What are the symptoms?	Non-specific systemic upset, irritability, malaise, fever. *Otalgia may not be the presenting feature*

Always examine a sick child's ears

What are the signs?	As above + bulging, injected, red TMs. The TM may burst under pressure, releasing fluid into the canal. Signs of complications should be excluded (below)
How is it treated?	**Supportive**: bed rest, analgesia, antipyretics, fluids **Specific**: oral antibiotics, eg amoxicillin, co-amoxiclav
What are the complications?	**Mastoiditis**: pain, tachycardia, high fever, fullness and tenderness just behind the ear ↓ **VII palsy**: usually settles after treatment ↓ **Meningitis**: irritability, headache, drowsiness, nausea, neck stiffness ↓ **Intracranial**: worsening confusion, venous sinus **abscesses** thrombosis, deterioration and death
How are these treated?	**Non-surgical**: admit, fluids, analgesia, IV antibiotics **Surgical**: *emergency mastoidectomy* or neurosurgical drainage

REFERRED EAR PAIN

What are the main *non-otological* causes of otalgia?	*Mnemonic:* the Ts: **T**onsillitis and other infections, eg parotitis, sinusitis **T**ooth decay **T**emporomandibular and C-spine joint disorders **T**umours of the head and neck

EAR DISCHARGE (OTORRHOEA)

Where can discharge originate?	The **external ear** (canal) and/or **middle ear**
What are the different types of otorrhoea and their likely causes?	**Purulent**: acute OE, acute OM **Mucoid**: chronic OM and perforation **Offensive**: chronic OM and cholesteatoma **Watery**: CSF leak (skull base #, post-op) **Bloody**: trauma (eg perforation, skull base #), and malignancy, eg SCC

CHRONIC SUPPURATIVE OTITIS MEDIA (CSOM)

What is CSOM?	CSOM is long-standing middle ear disease associated with TM perforation, discharge and hearing loss. It can be classified as **tubo-tympanic** or **attico-antral**
What is tubo-tympanic CSOM?	This involves a **central perforation of the TM** with **middle ear mucosal disease** (usually after acute OM which is slow to resolve). The patient has intermittent mucoid discharge and moderate conductive deafness, ie **safe** (no *major* complications)
What are treatment options?	**Aural toilet** for discharge: microsuction and drops **Hearing aids** for the conductive hearing loss **Repair of TM perforation**: prosthetic or fascia graft
What is attico-antral CSOM?	This is associated with **Eustachian tube dysfunction**, resulting in TM perforation or retraction. This produces **cholesteatomas**

What is a cholesteatoma? An abnormal nest of hyperkeratinising middle ear epithelium which destroys surrounding structures such as the ossicles and temporal bone, eroding into nerves and brain, ie **unsafe** if not treated.

The patient may have **offensive discharge**, **marked hearing loss** and **features of complications**

What are the treatment options? **Surgery** is usually required, involving excision of all the diseased tissue in the mastoid and middle ear (a mastoidectomy), to leave a **safe, dry** ear.

Regular follow-up will be necessary to check for recurrence

TRAUMA

What types of trauma can cause TM perforation? **Direct injury** (surgery, foreign body, eg cotton bud)

Indirect injury (barotrauma from slap across the ear, explosions, scuba diving, etc)

How is it managed? **Clinical examination** (of *both* ears!)

Hearing tests (clinical, PTA, tympanography) to exclude *gross* conductive deafness suggesting dislocation of the ossicles: a surgical emergency requiring immediate repair

Non-surgical: keep the ear **dry**, no drops or antibiotics required. Review at 2–3 weeks: a clean traumatic perforation will generally heal spontaneously

Surgical: repair of the perforation (unusual)

What are the features of skull base fractures?	**History**: *severe* blow to the temporo-parietal region (80%, producing a longitudinal #) or frontal region (20%, producing transverse #) **Clinical**: general condition (ABC and GCS), external manifestations (lacerations, Battle's sign, racoon eyes, facial palsy), CSF or blood otorrhoea, deafness (conductive and/or sensorineural), vertigo, CN IX/X/XI/XII injury
What are the principles of management?	**Head injury management** (see Chapter 11 Neurosurgery) **ENT management**: examination, prophylactic antibiotics, investigations (as for TM trauma) + CT temporal bones, CN VII decompression and repair of CSF leak if indicated

FACIAL PALSY

What are the branches of the facial nerve?	*Mnemonic:* **T**en **Z**ombies **B**u**ered **M**y **C**at **T**emporal **Z**ygomatic **B**uccal **M**andibular **C**ervical
How can you classify the causes of facial palsy?	The easiest way is to classify the causes is based on the **anatomy** of the complex course of the facial nerve (See Table 8.2)

PART III

Table 8.2

Intracranial section	1. CVA
	2. Brainstem tumour
	3. Acoustic neuroma (a Schwann cell tumour of CN VII)
Intratemporal section	1. Bell's palsy
	2. *Herpes zoster* infection (**Ramsay Hunt Syndrome**)
	3. Middle ear infection (acute or chronic)
	4. Trauma (esp. temporal bone #)
	5. Iatrogenic (surgical) injury
Extratemporal section	1. Iatrogenic (as in during parotidectomy)
	2. Facial lacerations
	3. Parotid tumours
General	1. Sarcoidosis
	2. Polyneuritis

What is the difference between upper and lower motor neurone facial palsy?

UMN (supranuclear): origin above the CN VII nucleus in the pons, forehead *spared,* eg CVA, brainstem tumour

LMN (infranuclear): origin below the VII nucleus, ipsilateral forehead *involved,* ie most other causes

How is facial palsy graded?

According to the **House–Brackmann** classification:

I   Normal function in all areas
II Mild dysfunction: seen on close inspection
III Moderate dysfunction: eye closure with effort
IV Moderate–severe: eye cannot be closed
V   Severe dysfunction: only flickers of movement
VI Total paralysis

What is Bell's palsy?

This is *idiopathic* facial paralysis and is a *diagnosis of exclusion*. The likely agent is a herpes virus infection, causing transient swelling and compression of VII. Many patients recover completely, but some will have residual weakness

What is Ramsay Hunt syndrome?

Comprises acute LMN VII paralysis and herpetic vesicular eruptions of the face, ear and mouth.
Other features include vertigo and sensorineural hearing loss. This is caused by *H. zoster* infection of the geniculate ganglion, affecting the adjacent VIII.
Weakness is often worse than in Bell's palsy and is less likely to recover

What is an acoustic neuroma?

This is a *rare* tumour of the Schwann cells of the VIIIth nerve at the cerebello-pontine angle. This can press on the intracranial portion of VII. It should be excluded (by MRI) in patients with unilateral hearing loss, tinnitus and/or VII palsy

What are the principles of treatment of VII palsy?

General management: reassurance, eye drops + patch, ophthalmological assessment and procedures, eg tarsorrhaphy if required. Investigation as needed
Specific management: according to cause. High dose steroids are useful for most causes, plus oral aciclovir for RHS and Bell's palsy. Further treatment and imaging with CT/MRI useful in cases of trauma, CVA and neoplasia

PART III

TINNITUS

What is tinnitus?

This is a sensation of sound which is *not* brought about by external stimuli (mechanical, acoustic or electrical). It affects most people at some stage, and may be *subjective* (heard by the patient only) or *objective* (audible to the examiner), eg carotid bruit

What causes tinnitus?

Local causes: *any* ear disease, cause of deafness (especially noise exposure and presbyacusis), ototoxic drugs and most types of ear surgery can cause tinnitus. Consider rare causes too, eg acoustic neuroma
General causes: Cardiovascular disease, hyperdynamic circulation, neurological causes, eg multiple sclerosis

How is it treated?

Mnemonic: **4Rs**

Reassurance: many cases resolve
Reversible causes: identify + treat, eg with hearing aid
Radio on low volume at night or noise generator
Referral to psychotherapist or counsellor

BALANCE DISORDERS

What is vertigo?

This is an **illusion of movement**, and is a cardinal feature of vestibular system disease

What organs influence balance?

Eyes (provide the majority of inputs)
Vestibular labyrinth (a smaller contribution)
Proprioceptors in muscle and joints
Cerebellum and **cerebrum** (the integration centres)

Balance disorders can arise from problems in any of these systems. The history will usually indicate the source. The causes can be **otological** or **non-otological**

What are the important points in the history of imbalance?	**General** health, social and ENT history **First attack**: precipitants, onset, duration **Periodicity** of attacks **Position** and **movements** during attacks **Relieving** or **preventative** factors **Hearing loss** **Tinnitus** **Co-existing medical problems** **Drugs** (prescribed and recreational) **Alcohol**
What are otological causes?	**Middle ear disease** (acute or chronic) **Trauma**, eg fractures, middle/inner ear surgery **Benign paroxysmal positional vertigo** (BPPV) **Labyrinthitis** **Ménière's disease** **Ototoxic drugs**, eg aminoglycosides **Tumours**, eg acoustic neuroma
What is BPPV?	This is vertigo which is **episodic** and **positional**, usually precipitated by certain movements such as head turning to one particular side, eg when lying down in bed. Attacks last for **seconds**, and fatigue with repeated movements

PART III

What causes BPPV?

Thought that small calcifications float in the semicircular canals (canaliths) and stimulate otoconia, which normally sense flow of canal fluid as the head moves, to adjust balance accordingly

How is it reproduced clinically?

With the **Dix–Hallpike manoeuvre**: from a sitting position, lie the patient down quickly, as you turn their head to one side, then repeat for the other side. One of these movements ought to precipitate an attack, and you should watch the eyes for nystagmus

How is it treated?

Many cases resolve spontaneously, but the **Epley manoeuvre** is often effective: repeat the Dix-Hallpike test to precipitate symptoms (30 s), then turn the head the *other* way (30 s). Then ask the patient to lie on *that* side, with the face pointing towards the floor (30 s). Then carefully sit the patient up over the edge of the bed, with the face pointing slightly downwards. This should displace the calcifications from the canals

What is labyrinthitis?

This is inflammation of the vestibular labyrinth, usually attributed to a viral infection. Vertigo lasts for **hours** or **days**, and may be associated with **sensorineural hearing loss** if the cochlea is involved

How is it treated?

Exclude other causes of imbalance. Vestibular sedatives, eg prochlorperazine, betahistine, antiemetics and IV fluids are useful, and acilovir can help in herpes-related cases. Vestibular exercises may be useful in the long term

What is Ménière's disease?	This affects young/middle-aged adults and comprises the following triad: 1. **Episodic vertigo** (minutes/hours) 2. **Tinnitus** 3. **Hearing loss** The patient is well between attacks
What causes it?	**Endolymphatic hydrops**, ie an expansion of the endolymphatic compartment occurs, but it is not known why
How is it treated?	**Support and sympathy** **Medical**: reduced dietary salt, vestibular sedatives, betahistine (a labyrinthine vasodilator), diuretics **Surgical**: grommet insertion (unproven) ± gentamicin drops (vestibulotoxic), endolymphatic sac decompression, section of the vestibular nerve
What are the non-otological anatomy causes of imbalance?	Consider the **history** and the The following can cause it: 1. Poor eyesight 2. Loss of proprioception, ie worse with age 3. Alcohol 4. Drugs 5. Cardiovascular disorders 6. Neurological disorders 7. CVA 8. Epilepsy 9. Head injury

NOSE

GENERAL CONCEPTS

How is the nose divided?	Into the **external nose**, the **nasal cavity** and the **paranasal sinuses**
Describe the parts of the external nose	Upper ⅓ *bony*: nasal bones, connect to the *nasion* at the forehead Lower ⅔ *cartilaginous*: alar cartilages and tip
Describe the nasal cavity	Stretches from vestibule (ant.) to nasopharynx (post.) **Septum** divides into left and right (composed of quadrilateral cartilage, perpendicular plate of ethmoid and vomer) **Lateral walls** have superior, middle and inferior turbinates (conchae), with meati below each. All lined with respiratory mucosa
Describe the paranasal sinuses	Air-filled, mucosa-lined cavities in the skull bones, extensions of the nasal cavity **Frontal**: develops in childhood, above orbit **Maxillary**: largest, between upper teeth and orbit **Ethmoid**: A and P, thin walled, in between orbits **Sphenoid**: next to int. carotid, III, cavernous sinus
Where do the sinuses drain?	All drain to nasal cavity to middle meatus *except:* 1. Sphenoid (sphenoethmoidal recess, superiorly) 2. Posterior ethmoid (superior meatus)

What is the blood supply of the nose?

Derived from the internal and external carotid aa.:
Ophthalmic a.→ant. and post. ethmoidal aa. (supplies region above middle turbinate)
Maxillary a.→sphenopalatine, palatine, labial aa. (supplies region below the middle turbinate)

What is Little's area?

A rich anastomotic region at the antero-inferior septum (branches of the ECA)

Why is it important?

This is the most common site of bleeding, where it can easily be seen and compressed

Figure 8.5 The arterial supply of the nose

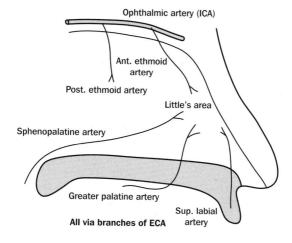

Ophthalmic artery (ICA)

Ant. ethmoid artery

Post. ethmoid artery

Little's area

Sphenopalatine artery

Greater palatine artery

Sup. labial artery

All via branches of ECA

Why is the venous drainage important?

The nose and midface drain via the facial and ophthalmic vv. into the **cavernous sinus**. This is a potential route for spread of apparently trivial infections

> **Investigate and treat infection of the midface and nose
> carefully – these can lead to cavernous sinus thrombosis,
> cranial nerve palsies (III, IV, VI) and fatal intracranial sepsis**

What should you ask about in the *nose* history?

Nose symptoms: obstruction, discharge, bleeding (epistaxis), change of smell
Associated symptoms: facial pain, otological symptoms, halitosis, neurological symptoms
General problems: allergies, asthma, medications, systemic disorders (eg arthritis), trauma, surgery, illicit drugs (cocaine)

How do you examine the nose?

Introduction: ask permission and if it's sore
Look at the patient's general condition and face
External nose: check alignment, profile, scars, etc
Internal nose: will require a headlight
1. *Push up tip of nose* gently with thumb and check the vestibule for discharge, obstruction, etc
2. *Anterior rhinoscopy*, using a Thuddichum's speculum on each side: visualise the inferior turbinate, then the middle and inferior meati above and below this. Remember the important structures draining into each (frontal/maxillary/ant. ethmoid sinuses into the middle meatus and the nasolacrimal duct into the inferior meatus)

3. *Nasendoscopy* (with rigid or flexible scopes) can visualise the areas not seen on anterior rhinoscopy. Pay particular attention to the postnasal space (where the Eustachian tube orifices lie)

Paranasal sinuses: palpate the overlying skin, check the teeth and eyes (movements and vision)

EPISTAXIS

What are the causes of epistaxis?

These can be divided into *local* and *general* causes:

Local:
1. Idiopathic (the commonest cause)
2. Trauma (nose picking, wiping, etc)
3. Infection (viral colds + nose blowing)
4. Iatrogenic (surgery)
5. Foreign body
6. Neoplasia

General:
1. Hypertension
2. Medications (aspirin, warfarin, etc)
3. Coagulopathies
4. Hereditary haemorrhagic telangiectasia (HHT; syn: **Osler–Weber–Rendu Syndrome**)

Where is the most likely source?

Little's area. It contains a rich arterial anastomosis *and* it is easily traumatised

What are the first aid measures?

1. **Basic Steps**: eye protection/apron/gloves
2. **ABC** and reassurance
3. Pinch nostrils tightly (>20 min)
4. Sit patient up and forwards
5. Ice pack on forehead/neck
6. Oxygen if necessary
7. IV access + fluids ± blood

PART III

What are the important historical points?

1. Details of current episode
2. Risk factors (see causes above)
3. Past history (general, ENT)
4. Drug history (in particular, anticoagulants)
5. Family history (ask about HHT)

What would you examine?

1. As for **ABC** (above)
2. General condition
3. Observations: RR, pulse, BP
4. Cardiovascular system
5. The nose
6. The throat (swallowed blood, blood trickling down from nasopharynx)

What investigations would you do?

Blood investigations:
1. FBC: Hb status
2. G&S: epistaxis can lead to life-threatening haemorrhage
3. Clotting: especially INR if on warfarin

How is it definitively managed?

As follows, each step being used if the preceding one fails:
1. Conservative (pinching, ice)
2. Cautery of bleeding point
3. Anterior/posterior nasal packing
4. Examination under GA with a view to surgery: artery ligation

---

Although frequently trivial and self-limiting, epistaxis can be a frightening event. In extreme cases it may be torrential and life-threatening

How do you cauterise the nose?

With the following steps:
1. Explain the procedure and reassure the patient
2. Use a nasal sucker *gently* to remove excess blood/clots from the nose and nasopharynx
3. Apply local anaesthetic spray to both nostrils
4. Apply Vaseline® around the nostrils to protect skin
5. Visualise the bleeding point
6. Use the sucker to keep the area clear
7. Press on the bleeding point gently with the tip of a silver nitrate stick – the bleeding will often settle
8. Check the nasopharynx is clear
9. Finally, apply nasal antibiotic cream to the nostrils

Do not use more than one silver nitrate stick

Do not cauterise both sides of the septum, to avoid perforation

Always use Vaseline® to protect the skin from the silver nitrate: this can stain permanently

---

How do you pack the nose?

With the following steps:
1. Explain the procedure and reassure the patient
2. Clear the blood/clots and anaesthetise the nose, as above
3. Choose a packing material: **nasal tampon** or **ribbon gauze**. Before insertion, remember that the nasal cavity is *large* and *>10 cm long*. The floor is *horizontal*

Both sides may require packing to achieve tamponade

What types of nasal packing material do you know of?

Nasal tampon, eg *Merocel®*: apply some nasal cream or lubricant and slide it carefully backwards and *horizontally* on the bleeding side. Ensure the anterior tip is inside the vestibule. Then apply some saline to the pack to allow it to swell

Ribbon gauze: use packing forceps to introduce a length of ribbon along the floor of the cavity to the postnasal space, then continue inserting ribbon in rows above this

---

Always secure the tampon or ribbon to the face with string/tape, to avoid posterior displacement and airway obstruction

---

What else should you do?

1. Leave the packs in for ≥24–48 hours and give low-dose oral antibiotics, eg Co-amoxiclav, to avoid infection/sinusitis
2. The patient should stay in hospital and *rest* + avoid hot food and drink throughout this period
3. Re-check FBC/clotting and correct any anomalies

What if these measures fail?

Re-evaluate ABC and resuscitate as appropriate. Consider examination under GA. The main options are **posterior packing** and **arterial ligation/embolisation**

How is posterior packing performed?

Posterior packing can be performed using the balloon of a Foley urinary catheter inflated in the postnasal space, with ribbon inserted around this, as above. Formal postnasal packs can also be used, held in place with tapes which are passed out through the nose

And ligation/embolisation?

Ligation or **embolisation** of the peripheral arteries (ethmoid, sphenopalatine, etc) may be required. In extreme cases the external carotid artery may be tied off

Is follow-up required?

Yes. Arrange nasendoscopy after the acute event: it is essential to exclude neoplasia as the cause of epistaxis

NASAL TRAUMA

List some important sequelae of nasal trauma.

Nasal injuries:
1. Nasal bone #
2. Septal fracture/dislocation
3. Septal haematoma/abscess
4. Epistaxis
5. Soft tissue injuries
6. Nasal lacerations

Local injuries:
1. **Airway compromise**
2. Head (brain) injury
3. Skull fractures/CSF leak
4. Facial fractures
5. Orbital fractures/eye injuries
6. Nerve injuries, eg infraorbital n.

Other injuries (usually concomitant as part of polytrauma):
1. C-spine fractures
2. Chest and abdominal injuries, etc

What are the principles of assessment?

ABC as for any injury. *Securing the airway (if deemed necessary) is the priority*

History:
1. Circumstances of injury
2. Time of injury
3. Loss of consciousness?
4. Progress since injury
5. Associated features, eg diplopia
6. Other current injuries
7. Previous injuries

Examination:

1. **ABCDE** as a priority
2. **Nose**: Shape, displacement, swelling, contours, profile, discharge (blood/CSF)
3. **Septum**: #/haematoma
4. **Orbits**: eye movements/vision, diplopia, orbital margins, infraorbital nerves
5. **Face**: swelling, fractures, lacerations, dental occlusion
6. **Other**: head, spine, chest, abdomen, limbs

What are the clinical features of nasal bone fractures?

Pain/tenderness, swelling around nasal bridge, haematoma, deformity of the nose, nasal obstruction, septal injury

Are radiographs necessary?

No. Nasal fracture is a **clinical** diagnosis

What are the principles of management?

1. Treat unsafe nasal injuries, eg septal haematoma
2. Correct the deformity to improve breathing and appearance (function and cosmesis). This is usually performed by manipulation (local or general anaesthetic) about 7–10 days after the injury

What is a septal haematoma?

A collection of blood beneath the mucoperichondrium of the septum. It usually follows trauma or septal surgery

What are the clinical findings?

Bilateral (or rarely unilateral) nasal obstruction, with a soft swelling arising from the septum and occluding the nasal passage(s)

Is this dangerous?

Yes. The blood supply of the cartilage is disrupted, causing cartilage necrosis and subsequent septal perforation ± collapse ± abscess ± saddle deformity of the nose. This is very difficult to correct

How is the haematoma managed?

Diagnosis: *Always* exclude a septal haematoma
Urgency: must be treated at once
Drainage: simple needle aspiration (small); formal incision and drainage (large)
Post-op: small drain in the cavity ± sutures ± nasal packing ± antibiotics

What is a septal abscess?

This is a collection of pus, clinically very much like a haematoma

And the management?

Similar to septal haematoma, but the infection must be treated aggressively to avoid intracranial spread

So what should be administered?

IV antibiotics for the infection, and heparin to prevent cavernous sinus thrombosis

What is CSF rhinorrhoea?

This is discharge of CSF from the nose. It can occur spontaneously, but most commonly follows injury of the **cribriform plate** by trauma or surgery

How is it diagnosed?

History: injury, ± continuous fluid leakage
Examination: clear fluid, signs of injury, altered sense of smell (olfactory nerve injury)
Special tests: check a sample of fluid for glucose and/or β_2-transferrin
Investigation: high resolution CT/endoscopy

How is it treated?	**Watch and wait**: small leaks may heal spontaneously **Antibiotics**: prophylaxis against meningitis, no proven benefits **Surgery**: fascia or prosthetic patch over defect

NASAL FOREIGN BODIES

How do nasal foreign bodies present?	Insertion **witnessed** or **admitted** by the patient (usually a young child) **Occult** insertion by child or **iatrogenic** insertion (eg ribbon gauze which is forgotten in the nose after surgery, etc). This usually presents with obstruction and *unilateral* offensive ± bloody nasal discharge ± discomfort
What is a rhinolith?	If presentation is delayed for months/years, the foreign body may act as a nidus for calcification: a **rhinolith**
What is the treatment of nasal foreign bodies?	There is a risk of aspiration and airway compromise, particularly in children. The object(s) should be removed *as soon as practical* with forceps or a wax hook, in clinic or under anaesthetic

RHINITIS

What is rhinitis?	Inflammation of the mucosal lining of the nose. It may be *allergic* or *non-allergic* (intrinsic)
What are the symptoms?	Nasal **obstruction**, **discharge** and **sneezing**. Allergic cases tend to follow exposure to allergens, and are often seasonal (pollen), while intrinsic cases are troublesome all year round

How is rhinitis treated?	**Avoid obvious allergens** as much as possible (eg carpets, feather pillows, pollen, pets) **Topical treatments** (sprays/drops): steroids (eg betamethasone, fluticasone), mast cell stabilisers (eg sodium chromoglicate which helps against sneezing) and topical decongestants (eg xylometazoline) **Systemic treatment** with antihistamines can reduce allergic symptoms and sneezing. Oral steroids are rarely used (side-effects) **Surgical treatment** is not often helpful. However, excision of large inferior turbinates and/or correction of septal deformities may reduce obstructive symptoms
What is rhinitis medicamentosa?	Rebound symptoms of rhinitis following the prolonged use of topical decongestants. These should be used sparingly and for short periods only (<1 week)

SINUSITIS

What is sinusitis?	Inflammation of the mucosal lining of the paranasal sinuses. It can be *acute* or *chronic*
What causes sinusitis?	Most cases are caused by **mucosal disease** of the nose itself or **structural abnormalities**, affecting mucus production and drainage. Disease in one sinus usually compromises the drainage and health of others

PART III

Other local predisposing factors include:

1. Nasal obstruction (eg from nasal packs)
2. Nasal trauma
3. Upper dental disease
4. Systemic factors, including general immunosuppression or debility (such as patients in intensive care)

What are the clinical features of acute sinusitis?

Symptoms:
1. Facial discomfort
2. Headache
3. Dental pain
4. Nasal obstruction
5. Nasal discharge
6. Foul smell (cacosmia)
7. Abscesses and eye complications

Signs:
1. Inflamed, discharging nose
2. Fever
3. General malaise
4. Periorbital swelling
5. Dental tenderness
6. Inflammatory markers

What are the potential complications?

1. Spread of infection to other sinuses and beyond
2. Generalised sepsis
3. Osteomyelitis
4. Orbital complications: periorbital cellulitis/abscess
5. Intracranial complications: extra-/sub-dural abscesses, meningitis, encephalitis, cerebral abscesses, death

Acute sinusitis and its complications may progress rapidly with dangerous consequences. It may occur in patients with no previous history and must be excluded as a source of sepsis (+ treated aggressively), particularly in the child or immunocompromised patient

What are the principles of management?

1. Early diagnosis
2. Treat the predisposing factor(s)
3. Treat the sinusitis
4. Treat the complications

Uncomplicated cases usually respond well to oral/topical decongestants ± analgesia ± broad spectrum antibiotics. Surgical drainage ± neurosurgical referral may be required for complicated cases

What is periorbital cellulitis?

This is most often seen in **children** following spread from ethmoid sinusitis. This can lead to a **subperiosteal abscess** and then to a **periorbital abscess**. *Vision is at critical risk*

What are the causes?

Mnemonic: **SIGHT**
Sinusitis
Insect bite
Glandular spread (eg dacrocystitis)
Haematological spread
Trauma

How do the symptoms/signs progress?

1. Erythema/oedema around the eye
2. Worsening oedema/eye closure
3. Loss of colour vision
4. Proptosis/diplopia
5. Loss of acuity
6. Loss of light reflex
7. Loss of vision
8. Neurological deterioration

PART III

What is the treatment?	1. High dose iv antibiotics 2. High resolution CT 3. ENT/ophthalmological emergency referral 4. Operative drainage as indicated by findings/scans
What are the features of chronic sinusitis?	Drainage and aeration of the sinuses are compromised, producing **nasal obstruction**, **facial discomfort**, **headaches**, chronic **nasal discharge**, **cacosmia** and **halitosis**
How is this treated?	**Medical management**, as for rhinitis, with topical and systemic therapy $\pm$ antibiotics **Surgical management** involves functional endoscopic sinus surgery (**FESS**). This aims to improve the aeration and drainage of the sinuses, thereby improving mucosal health

NASAL POLYPS

What are nasal polyps?	These are soft sacs of oedematous mucosa arising from the lining of the nose or sinuses (most often the ethmoid sinuses, from where they prolapse into the middle meatus). They are always bilateral
What are the associations?	1. **Chronic inflammation** of the nose from intrinsic/allergic/infective rhinitis or sinusitis 2. **Certain allergens** eg aspirin, NSAIDs 3. **Idiopathic** (a large proportion of cases) 4. **Neoplasia** should be considered in all cases, particularly with unilateral symptoms, pain and bloody discharge

5. **Other conditions** such as cystic fibrosis and bronchiectasis are associated, particularly in children with polyps

What are the symptoms?

Progressive nasal obstruction, which is usually **bilateral**. Nasal discharge, rhinitis, sinusitis and symptoms of associated conditions may also be present

What are the clinical signs?

Polyps which are small or high up in the nose may be difficult to see without an endoscope. Polyps are **grey**, and on palpation are soft, painless and do not bleed. Do not confuse these with prominent inferior turbinates (**pink**, firm and tender)

How are polyps treated?

Treat the underlying inflammatory process (with steroid nasal sprays, drops ± antibiotics)
Small polyps may regress spontaneously with medical treatment (a short course of oral steroids may help)
Large or resistant polyps ought to be excised endoscopically (and sent for histology). This is often combined with FESS, to improve the aeration and drainage of the sinuses

ADENOIDS

How do adenoids contribute to disease?

Adenoids can contribute to a number of disease processes, even if they are not enlarged. They lie in the postnasal space, and may therefore block the nasal airway ± Eustachian tubes and/or act as a sump for infection

PART III

What are the indications for adenoidectomy?

The most frequent indications for removal are:
1. Secretory otitis media (glue ear)
2. Chronic nasal obstruction/ discharge
3. Obstructive sleep apnoea (**OSA**)

Remember that adenoidectomy is never guaranteed to work, and the adenoids tend to atrophy by early teens in any case

THROAT

GENERAL CONCEPTS

What are the divisions of the 'throat'?

Oral cavity: buccal mucosa, alveoli (upper and lower), hard palate, ant. ⅔ of tongue, ant. tonsillar pillars

Nasopharynx: the area between the posterior choanae and the soft palate, containing the adenoids, Eustachian tube openings and fossae of Rosenmüller just medially (site of nasopharyngeal cancer)

Oropharynx: from soft palate to aryepiglottic folds, level with hyoid bone. Includes post. ⅓ of tongue, soft palate, tonsils and post. tonsillar pillars

Hypopharynx: continuation from oropharynx at level of hyoid, down to opening of oesophagus at level of cricoid cartilage

Larynx: system of cartilages (epiglottis, thyroid, cricoid and arytenoids), muscles and membranes. Divided into *supraglottis*, *glottis* (vocal cords) and *subglottis*

What are the major symptoms that can occur?

Pain (inflammation, infection, trauma, neoplasia)
Dysphagia/odynophagia (mechanical/functional)
Hoarseness (dysphonia)
Airway obstruction (stridor, foreign body, sleep apnoea)
Neck lumps/masses

How do you examine the throat?

1. **Introduction**: ask permission and if it's sore
2. Look at the patient's general condition and expose the face and neck
3. Sit in front of the patient with your legs *together* (don't straddle the patient!). Use a headlight or bull's eye lamp + head mirror to reflect the light
4. **Oral cavity/oropharynx**: full *inspection* of lips, tongue (all surfaces), buccal mucosa, salivary duct orifices, then use a tongue depressor to visualise the tonsillar arches, tonsils, soft palate and uvula. Then *palpate* the floor of mouth, tongue base and salivary glands/ducts for pain/swelling/stones
5. **Postnasal space**: this important site of pathology is examined via the nose with an endoscope or via the oropharynx using a postnasal mirror

PART III

6. **Laryngoscopy**: the larynx can be visualised *indirectly* using a laryngeal mirror or *directly* using a **flexible nasendoscope**. Inspect the tongue base, vallecula, epiglottis, posterior pharyngeal wall, pyriform fossae, arytenoids and true/false cords. Ask the patient to phonate/cough to assess cord movements

How do you examine the neck?

The neck should be examined systematically as part of any routine ENT or head and neck examination
Inspect for skin lesions, scars, lumps, tracheostomy, etc. Ask the patient to swallow some water and watch for thyroid movement, then ask them to count to 10 to assess the voice
Palpate the neck *from behind*. Examine each lymph node region with the pulps of the fingers in an orderly sequence, eg submental, then submandibular and mastoid/preauricular nodes (and parotid glands), moving up to the occipital nodes. Then move down the sternomastoid to the jugular notch and up to the paratracheal nodes and thyroid. Finally, check the supraclavicular fossa and posterior triangle. Cervical lymph nodes are generally grouped into 5 levels (see Figure 8.6)

Figure 8.6

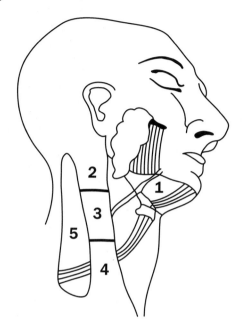

SORE THROAT

What are the main causes sore throat?

Consider the **anatomy** and/or the **of aetiology**:

Pharynx	Infection
Tonsils	Inflammation
Larynx	Trauma
Epiglottis	Neoplasia

For example, acute pharyngitis, tonsillitis, glandular fever, laryngitis, epiglottitis, deep space neck infections, lymphoma, laryngeal cancer, etc

The *history* and *age* of the patient will usually limit the differential diagnoses

PHARYNGITIS

What are the features of pharyngitis?

Erythema and soreness of the pharyngeal mucosa, usually in the context of a URTI

What organisms are responsible?

The cause is usually **viral**, although streptococcal infections are sometimes seen (more painful, associated fevers, mucopus)

What is the treatment?

Most cases settle with rest, fluids and simple analgesia. Oral antibiotics may be required

TONSILLITIS

Who gets tonsillitis?

Typically seen in children and young adults. *Can* occur in older people, but always consider another cause of sore throat, eg laryngitis, neoplasia

What are the symptoms?

Patients with tonsillitis are usually systemically unwell ± febrile, with tender cervical lymphadenopathy and **odynophagia**. The tonsils are red ± enlarged ± exudates in the **tonsillar crypts**

What organisms cause tonsillitis?

Many cases are viral. Streptococci are the most common bacterial cause

How is tonsillitis treated?

Bed rest, fluids and good analgesia ± oral antibiotics

Which antibiotics?

Oral penicillin V is the first-line antibiotic (works well against streptococci)

Which antibiotic should be avoided?

Amoxicillin! May precipitate a nasty rash if the patient in fact has glandular fever

Is admission ever necessary?

Admission for iv fluids ± antibiotics will be necessary for patients with airway obstruction or inability to swallow fluids/medications

What are the possible complications?	**Local**:
	1. Airway obstruction
	2. Absolute dysphagia
	3. Deep space neck infections/ abscess formation (peritonsillar, parapharyngeal, retropharyngeal)
	Systemic:
	1. Septicaemia
	2. Meningitis
	3. Acute rheumatic fever
	4. Glomerulonephritis

PERITONSILLAR ABSCESS (QUINSY)

What is a quinsy?	A **peritonsillar abscess** (PTA)
What are the features of a PTA?	The following:
	1. Existing attack of acute tonsillitis, with worsening **unilateral** pain and swelling around the tonsil
	2. Inability to speak properly (**hot potato voice**)
	3. Inability to swallow properly (they may be **drooling**)
	4. Inability to open mouth fully (**trismus** due to pterygoid irritation)
	5. Examination reveals gross deviation of the uvula and palate to the contralateral side
How can they be remembered?	*Mnemonic:* **MOST FIT**
	Muffled voice
	Odynophagia
	Swelling (peritonsillar!)
	Trismus
	Fetid odour
	Inflammation (peritonsillar)
	Temperature rise

PART III

How is PTA treated?

1. Admit
2. **Drainage** of the abscess with needle/syringe
3. IV fluids
4. Analgesia
5. IV (then oral) antibiotics
6. One dose of steroids (dexamethasone)

What about para-/retro-pharyngeal abscesses?

These can follow on from tonsillitis/PTA or from simple URTIs, particularly in children. They are **surgical emergencies**, as the *airway* is at risk *and* infection may track into the *mediastinum*

What is the management?

After securing the **airway**, admit for **iv antibiotics ± drainage**

Suspect deep space neck infections in the patient with existing tonsillitis or URTI, with subsequent worsening systemic upset, dysphagia and/or stridor

---

INFECTIOUS MONONUCLEOSIS (GLANDULAR FEVER)

What is glandular fever?

Also known as infectious mononucleosis (IM), and tends to affect teenagers and adults. It is caused by Epstein–Barr virus (EBV)

How is IM different from tonsillitis?

Onset is more gradual, typically with greater malaise, gross cervical lymphadenopathy and more obvious **tonsillar exudates**

How is it diagnosed?

Paul–Bunnell (monospot) blood test: looks for abnormal lymphocytes

What is the danger of IM?

EBV can cause a transient hepatitis and splenomegaly. Always examine abdomen for hepatosplenomegaly if IM is suspected. Also do LFTs

How is IM managed?

Treatment is the same as for tonsillitis, but antibiotics have no benefit. *Examine the abdomen to exclude hepatosplenomegaly*

What advice should be given to patients?

Avoid contact sports for ≥6 weeks to avoid liver or spleen injuries

What are the indications for tonsillectomy?

The only **absolute** indications for tonsillectomy are:
1. Suspected neoplasia
2. Frank airway obstruction
3. Tonsillitis, *more than five* episodes per year for two *consecutive* years *or* if it interferes grossly with education or work
4. Previous PTA (quinsy): most often done after *two* abscess episodes
5. Obstructive sleep apnoea (OSA): large tonsils ± adenoids can worsen breathing, especially at night

DYSPHAGIA

What is the difference between *dysphagia* and *odynophagia*?

Dysphagia is difficultly in swallowing, **odynophagia** refers to pain on swallowing

What are the important features in a *dysphagia* history?

The history should be directed towards the likely causes, remembering that poor flow through any viscus or vessel can be attributed to **intraluminal**, **mural**, or **extramural** causes:
Acute dysphagia (food bolus *obstruction*, *CVA*, inflammation, deep neck *infections*) or **chronic**? Problems with the **action of swallowing** suggest a **neuromuscular** problem: ask also about **speech problems**

PART III

Regurgitation of unaltered food ± gurgling in the neck ± aspiration suggests a **pharyngeal pouch** (elderly patients) or **achalasia** (younger patients)

Increasing dysphagia to foods *then* fluids suggests a mechanical stricture eg **neoplasia**

Associated symptoms such as pain, weight loss, otalgia, hoarseness and/or neck lump also suggest possible *neoplasia*

Swallowed foreign body, eg fish bone, piece of meat, etc. Onset of symptoms immediately or soon after ingestion. Varying degrees of dysphagia ± dysphonia depending on site and type. Fish bones usually stick into the **tonsil** and so usually visible O/E, but often radiolucent. Larger objects tend to lodge at cricopharyngeus (level of C6). Try iv fluids, Buscopan® ± diazepam. May need endoscopic removal

Globus pharyngeus (sensation of a 'lump in the throat') may be psychogenic, but a physical cause (eg reflux laryngitis or neoplasia) should be excluded

How is dysphagia investigated?

This should be directed by the **history** and full ENT and systemic **examination**

An outpatient **barium swallow** will outline the hypopharynx and oesophagus very well, and is sensitive, cheap and quick. Formal rigid **laryngoscopy/oesphagoscopy + biopsy** (in theatre, under GA) is the gold standard, but this is usually reserved for those cases where neoplasia is more likely

DYSPHONIA

What is the difference between *dysphonia* and *aphonia*?	**Dysphonia** refers to an alteration in voice quality, whereas **aphonia** is reserved for total loss of voice
How is dysphonia classified?	It can be **organic** or **non-organic** (See Table 8.3).

Table 8.3 Organic causes (mechanical)

Inflammation/infection	Laryngitis – acute or chronic (reflux, smoking, etc)
Neoplasia*	Laryngeal cancer, laryngeal papillomatosis (HPV infection)
Systemic disease	Hypothyroidism, rheumatoid disease
Neurological disorder	eg CVA, bulbar palsy, myasthenia gravis, etc
Non-organic causes (functional)	
Overactivity	Nodules – excessive voice use
Habitual dysphonia	Abnormal patterns of voice production, can be stress-related
Psychogenic dysphonia	No laryngeal disease present, often due to depression, anxiety, neuroses

How is dysphonia investigated?	This is directed by the **history** and **examination**. **Flexible endoscopy** is a useful first-line measure in clinic, but the investigation of choice is **rigid laryngoscopy ± biopsy** (under GA, in theatre).

---

* **Hoarseness with no obvious precipitant, lasting more than 3 weeks, is caused by laryngeal cancer until proven otherwise. ENT referral for direct laryngoscopy is mandatory**

How is dysphonia managed?	**Organic** dysphonias may respond to treatment of the underlying cause, while *non-organic* examples may respond well to speech and language therapy and/or psychotherapy

AIRWAY OBSTRUCTION

What is *stridor*?	**Noisy breathing** caused by partial obstruction of the respiratory tract ***at or below the larynx***
What is *stertor*?	**Noisy breathing** caused by partial obstruction of the respiratory tract ***above the larynx***
What are the causes of airway obstruction?	Remember that obstruction of *any* tube, vessel or viscus can result from **luminal**, **mural**, or **extramural** causes. Also consider *anatomy*, the *age group* involved and whether *congenital* or *acquired*. See Table 8.4

Table 8.4 Neonates (congenital)

Choanal atresia or other causes of nasal obstruction
Craniofacial abnormalities, large tongue, etc
Neurological abnormalities (floppy nasopharynx)
Laryngomalacia
Subglottic stenosis
Children
Laryngotracheitis (croup)
Foreign body
Acute epiglottitis
Acute tonsillitis/large tonsils
Deep space neck infections
Adults
Laryngeal cancer
Laryngitis
Supraglottitis/epiglottitis
Foreign body
Laryngotracheal trauma

What are the signs of airway obstruction?	1. **Tachycardia**
	2. **Tachypnoea** (*or* bradypnoea/ bradycardia *in extremis*)
	3. Audible stridor
	4. Dysphonia
	5. Inability to complete sentences
	6. Use of accessory muscles of respiration
	7. Nasal flaring
	8. Tracheal tug
	9. Intercostal/subcostal recession of chest wall

EPIGLOTTITIS

What is epiglottitis?	An uncommon, but life-threatening, infection of the larynx and supraglottis (particularly the epiglottis)
What is the responsible organism?	*Haemophilus influenzae* type B is the most common cause
Who gets it?	Young children are most often affected, but adults can develop supraglottitis too
How can it be prevented?	HiB vaccination is believed to have reduced its incidence, but it is still seen
What are the clinical features?	*Know this cold!* It starts as a **sore throat** which worsens, accompanied by **malaise** and **high fever**. The child becomes **dysphonic** and **odynophagic**, eventually **unable to swallow saliva**. **Stridor** and fatal airway obstruction may intervene rapidly

PART III

How is epiglottitis managed?

Know this cold as well!!

The diagnosis should be obvious
The airway is at *critical risk*

1. Do *nothing* to frighten the child, as this could precipitate stridor and airway obstruction; nurse in a quiet area with mother present
2. Do *not* examine the child's throat: again, this could precipitate stridor and airway obstruction
3. *No* blood tests or X-rays are needed
4. Call a senior (paediatric) anaesthetist to intubate the child as a *priority*
5. Inform senior ENT in case intubation fails and tracheostomy is needed
6. Transfer to ITU
7. Administer IV antibiotics

What are the antibiotics of choice?

Cefuroxime (3rd generation cephalosporin)
Chloramphenicol can also be used

CROUP

What is croup?

Viral laryngotracheobronchitis

Who gets it?

Commonly seen in young children

What are the symptoms?

Characterised by moderate systemic upset and a **barking cough**

What are the risks?

Respiratory distress and dangerous airway obstruction may occur

What is the management?

Symptoms usually settle with O_2 + nebulised steroids $\pm$ nebulised adrenaline

INHALED FOREIGN BODY

What are the clinical features of foreign body inhalation?

History:
1. Witnessed event
2. Eating small food items, eg peanuts
3. Bout of coughing/choking
4. Past history of foreign body
5. Occult event + delayed presentation

Examination: *Child may be entirely well*

Tachycardia → tachypnoea → respiratory distress

May present with collapse and apnoea

Chest: wheeze ± hyperinflated or collapsed

What are the possible X-ray findings?

Chest films (PA and lateral) are essential to rule out life-threatening respiratory problems (eg pneumothorax) immediately

1. Film may look entirely normal
2. A radio-opaque foreign body may be seen
3. The lung field(s) *distal* to the obstruction may be **hyperinflated** (**emphysematous**) or **collapsed/ consolidated**
4. The object may act as a 'ball-valve', allowing *inspired* air past it, but blocking *expiration*, causing hyperinflation
5. Alternatively, the object may block all airflow, causing distal absorption of O_2 and collapse ± consolidation

PART III

What are the principles of management?

1. **Basic steps**: ABCDE
2. **Heimlich manoeuvre** as necessary
3. **Intubation** if *in extremis*
4. History and examination (if time)
5. Locate the site of obstruction (X-rays)
6. Arrange extraction (with bronchoscope, under GA) by an ENT specialist as soon as practical

UPPER AIRWAY TRAUMA

What are the mechanisms of laryngotracheal trauma?

The airway may be injured by insults from **within** or **without** the lumen.
Within:
1. Endotracheal intubation (iatrogenic)
2. Inhalation of smoke/hot air from a fire/corrosive agents. In these cases, the history and examination (charred lips/nostrils, facial burns, sooty sputum, etc) are vital

Without:
1. Blunt injuries, eg RTA, sport
2. Penetrating trauma, eg knife wounds.

What are the presenting features?

1. Pain from the neck
2. Dysphonia
3. Odynophagia
4. Stridor and respiratory distress
5. Bleeding from the airway or skin
6. Features of other related injuries eg C-spine, chest (pneumothorax), cardiac, head, etc

> The presentation may be *delayed* and *catastrophic* – always *pre-empt* sudden respiratory compromise in patients with any history of possible airway injury. Consult a senior anaesthetist ± ENT specialist *at once* to secure the airway

SECURING THE AIRWAY

What basic life support (BLS) measures can improve the airway?

Manoeuvres: position the patient with neck slightly flexed and head extended ('sniffing the morning air') ± chin lift ± jaw thrust
Bag and mask ventilation is usually very effective
Adjuncts: oropharyngeal (Guedel) and nasopharyngeal airways

> Always be aware of possible C-spine injury, and re-assess the airway after each manoeuvre

What are the indications for securing the airway?

The airway is *unsafe* or *potentially* unsafe in a number of circumstances. Intervention may be planned (elective) or unplanned (emergency). The secured airway will allow airflow and gas exchange *and* protect the distal tracheobronchial tree from further insults
Planned, eg for general anaesthesia, gradual or anticipated respiratory compromise (eg on ICU)
Unplanned, eg airway infections (epiglottitis), asthma, foreign bodies, trauma, tumours, etc

PART III

What methods are available?	**Endotracheal intubation**, via *oro*tracheal or *naso*tracheal routes

Endotracheal intubation, via *oro*tracheal or *naso*tracheal routes

Tracheostomy, performed percutaneously in ICU (elective) or surgically (elective or emergency) Useful for patients with upper airway obstruction or trauma, or when prolonged intubation is necessary in ICU

Cricothyroidotomy, by passing a needle through the cricothyroid membrane. Limited *jet* ventilation is then possible. Useful to *buy time* for the patient *in extremis*, but the airway is *not* secure

---

For patients with respiratory compromise, the immediate priority is *ventilation* and *oxygenation*

BLS manoeuvres, adjuncts and bag/mask ventilation are effective and easily performed. Advanced techniques are reserved for specialists with appropriate training

---

HEAD AND NECK

NECK LUMPS

How do you classify neck lumps?	Acute vs chronic

Acute vs chronic
Painful vs painless
Stable vs enlarging vs regressing
Benign vs malignant (primary/secondary)
Congenital vs acquired
Localised vs systemic disorder
Midline vs lateral
Anterior triangle Submandibular glands, parotid tail, thyroid, larynx, lymph nodes, carotids
Posterior triangle Supraclavicular nodes, XI

What are the causes of cervical lymphadenopathy?

As with most other neck lumps, nodes can become enlarged for several reasons:

1. **Infection** (eg after tonsillitis, IM, URTI, TB)
2. **Inflammation** (eg sarcoidosis)
3. **Neoplasia** (primary/secondary)
4. **Congenital**
5. **Idiopathic**

History and examination will be centred around eliciting one of these causes

What are the investigations?

Will ultimately depend on the cause, but *generally*:

Blood investigations:

1. FBC ($\uparrow$ WBC in infection)
2. ESR ($\uparrow$ in conditions such as sarcoidosis, TB)
3. CRP (inflammatory marker, but non-specific)

Imaging:

1. Ultrasound $\pm$ fine needle aspiration (FNA)
2. MRI neck $\pm$ CT chest for diagnosis/staging of neoplasia

Operative investigation:

1. Excision biopsy of node(s)
2. Panendoscopy of upper aerodigestive tract to find a primary mass

PART III

DEVELOPMENTAL ABNORMALITIES

What are the derivatives of the branchial arches?	Use this great mnemonic: ***Mnemonic:*** **M**uscles **S**upport the **P**harynx and **L**arynx 1st Arch (**M**andibular arch): Also known as **M**eckel's cartilage **M**uscles of **m**astication **M**andible **M**andibular nerve (CN V$_3$) **M**ucous membrane (anterior ⅔ of tongue) **M**axillary artery 2nd Arch (Hyoid arch): **S**tapes **S**tyloid process **S**tylohyoid ligament **S**uperior part and lesser horn of hyoid bone **S**miling muscles (muscles of facial expression) and their nervous supply (CN VII) 3rd Arch: Stylo**pharyngeus** muscle Glosso**pharyngeus** muscle Inferior part and greater horn of hyoid bone 4th & 6th Arches: The **larynx**: Cartilages of the **larynx**: thyroid, cricoid, aretynoid, epiglottis Muscles of the **larynx** Pharyngeal and **laryngeal** parts of the vagus nerve (CN X) 5th Arch: no derivatives
What are the common developmental neck lumps?	**Midline**: 1. Thyroglossal cyst 2. Dermoid cyst 3. Thyroid mass

Lateral:
1. Cervical node
2. Branchial cyst
3. Cystic hygroma
4. Haemangioma
5. Malignancy

What is a thyroglossal cyst?

This is the most common midline mass. It is a midline neck swelling representing a cystic swelling of an otherwise non-patent thyroglossal tract

Where is it found?

Usually just below the hyoid bone, although it can develop anywhere along the embryonic thyroglossal duct, between the foramen caecum of the tongue and the thyroid gland

How does it present?

As a lump which moves up with tongue protrusion. It may also become infected and present as a neck abscess or a pus-draining sinus

How is it investigated?

With USS, to delineate the anatomy *and* to demonstrate a normal thyroid gland as the cyst may be the only site of active thyroid tissue. If excised in this situation, the patient will be rendered hypothyroid

How is it managed?

Via **excision**: involves removal of the cyst, tract and *central portion of the hyoid*, to reduce recurrence (**Sistrunk's procedure**)

What is a dermoid cyst?

A remnant of embryonic fusion, almost always found in the midline. It may become enlarged or infected

How is it investigated?

With USS ± MRI, as it may extend intracranially, with implications for excision

What is a branchial cyst?

A cyst related to abnormalities of a branchial arch, usually the **second**

PART III

201

Who gets it?	It tends to present in late childhood as a swelling **just anterior to the sternomastoid**. It may become infected
How is it treated?	It can be left alone if asymptomatic. Excision should include the cyst itself ± any tracts extending deeper
What is a cystic hygroma?	A mass or abnormally dilated lymphatic channels, usually presenting as a soft mass at birth. It is characteristically **brilliantly transilluminable**
How is it treated?	Treatment is usually delayed for several months, to allow the child to grow (unless there are airway risks); it consists of sclerosant injections and/or excision
What is a haemangioma?	A benign capillary tumour, which enlarges rapidly after birth (**strawberry naevus**). It usually regresses spontaneously during childhood
How is it treated?	It is left alone, unless blocking vision or the airway

ADULT NECK LUMPS

How are these categorised?	Again, lumps can be **midline** or **lateral**
What are the commonest _midline_ lumps?	**Benign thyroid lumps:** 1. Diffuse goitre (physiological or low iodine). 2. Multinodular goitre (toxic or non-toxic) 3. Single nodule

Thyroid neoplasia:
1. Adenoma
2. Papillary Ca (75%): lymphatic spread, good 5-year survival rate
3. Follicular Ca (15%): haematogenous spread, mets
4. Medullary Ca: association with MEN II syndromes
5. Anaplastic Ca: elderly patients, grim prognosis
6. Lymphoma (rare, treated with radio-/chemotherapy)

Thyroglossal/dermoid cysts

What are the commonest *lateral* lumps?

1. Lymph nodes
2. Salivary glands (inflammation/ neoplasia).
3. Vascular masses, eg carotid aneurysm

INFECTION

Where are the main sites of head/neck infection?

Mouth:
1. Salivary glands (**sialadenitis**, known as **parotitis** if affecting the parotid gland)
2. Floor of mouth (**Ludwig's angina**)
3. Gums (**Vincent's angina**)

Throat:
1. Tonsillitis
2. PTA (quinsy)
3. Other deep space neck infections (eg retro- and parapharyngeal abscesses)
4. Lymph nodes (**lymphadenitis**)

Nose: nasal and paranasal sinus sepsis

Airway:
1. Supraglottitis/epiglottitis
2. Laryngitis
3. Tracheitis

Skin: cutaneous abscesses, cellulitis

What type of infection is Ludwig's angina?	Streptococcal
What type of infection is Vincent's angina?	Spirochetal

NEOPLASIA

What are the main types of head and neck cancer?	The majority of malignancies are **squamous cell carcinomas** (SCC). Adenocarcinoma, lymphoma and other rarer malignancies are sometimes seen in specific sites, eg salivary glands, thyroid, etc **Skin cancers** (SCC, BCC, melanoma) should also be considered
What aetiological factors are involved?	See Table 8.5

Table 8.5

Tumour	Aetiological agent
SCC: Oral Lingual Tonsillar Laryngeal Pharyngeal	**Smoking** **Alcohol** Age Male sex Poor oral hygiene Diet (eg betel/tobacco chewing) Premalignant conditions eg leukoplakia
Thyroid Ca	**Radiation exposure**
Nasopharyngeal Ca	Salted fish Childhood EBV infection
Lymphomas Kaposi sarcoma	**Immunosuppressed states** eg HIV, post-transplant, etc
Hypopharyngeal Ca	Chronic iron deficiency (Patterson–Brown–Kelly syndrome)

How can the classic signs for nasopharyngeal carcinoma be remembered?	*Mnemonic:* **NOSE** **N**eck mass **O**bstructed nasal passage **S**erous otitis media (usually unilateral) **E**pistaxis or discharge
What are the major symptoms of head and neck cancers?	For *any* cancer, the symptoms can be divided into: **General symptoms of malignant disease** eg weight loss, weakness, lethargy **Effects of local disease** eg pain, lump, compression, ulceration **Effects of metastatic disease** eg pathological fractures, liver failure, etc **Paraneoplastic syndromes** eg hypercortisolaemia due to ACTH secretion by small cell lung cancers (See also Table 8.6)

Table 8.6

General symptoms	Pain Cosmetic changes Head/neck swellings Speech problems Mastication problems Swallowing problems Weight loss Reduced appetite Co-existing conditions Features of metastatic disease
Oral cancer	Chronic ulcer Metastatic neck node Pain (less common) Halitosis

Continued

PART III

Table 8.6 *Continued*

Tonsillar cancer	Unilateral tonsil enlargement Pain (referred otalgia) Recurrent tonsillitis/quinsy Metastatic neck node
Salivary gland cancers	Swelling and cosmetic effects Blockage of ducts/infection Metastatic neck node Pain Nerve compression, eg VII
Thyroid cancers	Midline neck swelling Metastatic neck node
Hypopharyngeal cancer	Dysphagia Dysphonia Metastatic neck node
Laryngeal cancer	Dysphonia (if glottic) ? No symptoms (if subglottic) Metastatic neck node Dysphagia Pain
Lymphoma	Neck nodes Other nodes 'B' symptoms: weight loss, low grade pyrexia, night sweats

What is paramount in head and neck cancer?

Early evaluation:

1. **History** and **examination**: should be exhaustive, covering the head and neck *and* the other systems. Many head and neck cancers are occult for long periods, and early detection has a crucial effect on prognosis and treatment options

2. **Referral to a specialist centre**, ideally within two weeks of the original presentation

What diagnostic tools are used?

Diagnosis: the following tests are used in combination for **diagnosis** of the primary tumour and **staging** information to guide treatment:

1. **USS** of the offending mass/lesion, usually **FNA** for cytological analysis
2. **MRI** of the neck: shows soft tissue detail very clearly; important in the identification of local tumour spread and nodal metastases
3. **CT chest**, to exclude distant metastatic disease: this would rule out attempting curative surgery
4. **PET** (positron emission tomography) of the head/neck: highlights areas of high metabolic activity (eg tumour masses) and is particularly useful when trying to identify an undiagnosed primary in a patient with nodal disease
5. **Examination under anaesthetic ± biopsy** is essential, allowing evaluation of the tumour(s) *and* a formal tissue sample for histology

Who need to be involved in planning treatment?

Planning: all patients with head and neck cancers should be discussed by a **multi-disciplinary team**. This includes:

1. Surgeon
2. Radiologist
3. Pathologist
4. Oncologist
5. Nurse specialist (Macmillan)
6. Speech and language therapist

PART III

What are the treatment options?

The available options include:

1. **Surgery** (curative vs non-curative)
2. **Radiotherapy** (primary or adjuvant, after surgery)
3. **Chemotherapy** (largely limited to lymphomas)
4. **Palliative care** (with Macmillan nurse specialists)

CHAPTER 9: OPHTHALMOLOGY

CLINICAL ANATOMY

Figure 9.1

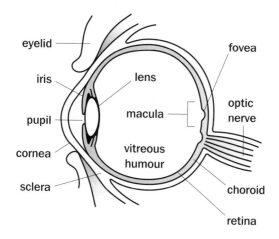

THE PUPIL

What are the light reflexes?	**Direct** (constrict when light shown directly over it) or **consensual** (constrict when light shown on other eye)
What controls the afferent limb?	Optic nerve (CN2)
And the efferent limb?	Parasympathetic fibres on the oculomotor (CN3)
What afferent defect do you know of?	Absent direct reflex due to optic nerve (neuritis or atrophy) or diffuse retinal pathology. Consensual reflex would be intact; when swinging light from good to bad eye, the bad eye will dilate

What efferent defect do you know of?	Due to oculomotor nerve pathology. If painful, always consider posterior communicating artery aneurysm. Other causes include cavernous sinus lesion, diabetes and space-occupying lesions (pupil fibres run peripherally in the CN3, therefore affected first in compressive lesions)
What is the Argyll Robertson pupil?	Meiosis (small pupil), constricts on accommodation but not to light. Causes include syphilis and diabetes *Mnemonic:* prostitute analogy – accommodates but does not react
What is the Holmes–Adie pupil?	Dilated pupil, occurs in the young, classic vermiform (worm-like) movement on reaction to light. **Holmes–Adie syndrome** if knee and ankle jerks are also absent
What is Horner's syndrome?	Partial ptosis, enophthalmos, meiosis ± anhidrosis (absent sweating) due to disruption of the sympathetic supply of the face

RED EYE

How can this be classified?	Into painful and painless: **Painful**: Acute angle closure glaucoma (AACG) Conjunctivitis Keratitis Episcleritis Scleritis Anterior uveitis Corneal abrasion/foreign body (FB) **Painless**: Subconjunctival haemorrhage Conjunctivitis (can also be painful) Blepharitis (can also be painful) Dry eye syndrome (can also be painful)

How can the causes of red eye be easily remembered?	*Mnemonic:* **GO SUCK** **G**laucoma **O**cular trauma (FB, abrasion, haemorrhage) **S**cleritis **U**veitis **C**onjunctivitis **K**eratitis

CONJUNCTIVITIS

What is it?	Inflammation of the conjunctiva
What are the causes?	Bacterial Viral Allergic Chlamydial
How does it present?	**Bacterial:** *Signs:* purulent discharge, papillae present *Investigation:* conjunctival swab *Treatment:* controversial evidence on treatment before positive culture; chloramphenicol qds for 5 days **Viral:** *Symptoms:* photophobia, FB sensation, starts in one eye and spreads to the other within a few days *Signs:* watery discharge, conjunctival follicles, pre-auricular lymph nodes (history of recent URTI) *Treatment:* artificial tears, frequent handwashing *Outcome: very* contagious; can get worse 4–7 days after onset; may not resolve for 2–3 weeks

PART III

Allergic:
Symptoms: itchy, watery discharge, history of atopy
Signs: red oedematous eyelids, chemosis, conjunctival papillae
Treatment: artificial tears, antihistamine, topical steroid (only by ophthalmologist!)

KERATITIS

What is it?	Corneal inflammation (characterised by white corneal infiltrate)
What is the aetiology?	Bacterial Viral Also fungal
What predisposes to bacterial keratitis?	Contact lens wear Trauma Pre-existing corneal pathology
How does bacterial keratitis present?	**Bacterial**: *Symptoms*: painful, red, watery eye; FB sensation; photophobia; blurred vision *Signs*: conjunctival injection (often circumcorneal); corneal infiltrate (white lesion); Fluorescein staining around or in the base of the lesion *Investigation*: corneal scrape; send for Gram stain, culture and sensitivities *Treatment*: broad-spectrum topical antibiotics until sensitivities available, eg ciprofloxacin drops hourly with daily review

And viral?

Depends on the type. There are 2 types: HSV 1 *Herpes zoster*

Herpes simplex 1 (HSV1):

Symptoms: can be a primary infection in childhood, or reactivation in adults. Symptoms of a viral illness usually prevail

Signs (primary infection): skin/lid vesicles, preauricular lymphadenopathy, conjunctivitis

Signs (reactivation): classic **dendritic ulcer** (stains with fluorescein)

Treatment: topical aciclovir ointment × 5/day

Herpes zoster ophthalmicus (HZO, shingles):

Aetiology: caused by reactivation of *Varicella zoster* virus and migration down the sensory fibres of the ophthalmic branch of the trigeminal nerve (CN Va)

Symptoms: usually elderly or immunocompromised preherpetic neuralgia. Vesicular skin rash

Signs: keratitis, conjunctivitis, cranial nerve palsies

Treatment: oral aciclovir

EPISCLERITIS

What is it?

Inflammation of the episclera (layer of tissue between conjunctiva and sclera)

What is the most common cause?

Most commonly idiopathic

How does it present?	*Symptoms*: red eye, mildly painful, typically in young adults *Signs*: sectorial redness in one eye; engorged vessels (larger then conjunctival vessels); blanching with phenylephrine 2.5% drops *Treatment*: artificial tears

SCLERITIS

What is it?	Inflammation of scleral vessels
What is the aetiology?	50% have **associated systemic disease**, eg rheumatoid arthritis, Wegener's granulomatosis, SLE, inflammatory bowel disease
How does it present?	*Symptoms*: painful red eye which wakes patient from sleep and may radiate to the forehead Insidious drop in vision *Signs*: inflamed scleral, episcleral and conjunctival vessels. Scleral vessels do *not* blanch with phenylephrine *Treatment*: ophthalmology review for dilated fundal exam and *investigation for other systemic illness*

ANTERIOR UVEITIS

What is it?	Inflammation of the anterior uvea (iris + ciliary body)
What is its aetiology?	The following: 1. Idiopathic 2. HLA B27 associated 3. Trauma 4. Infective 5. Drug-induced

How does it present?

Symptoms: painful red watery eye, photophobia, blurred vision
Signs: circumcorneal congestion (**ciliary flush**), corneal precipitates, small pupil (due to posterior synechiae; iris adhesion to lens capsule)
Treatment: refer to ophthalmologist for dilated fundal exam, IOP check. Topical steroids (prednisolone 1%) and dilation of the fundus to break the synechiae (cyclopentolate 1%)

CORNEAL ABRASION/FOREIGN BODY

How does it present?

As a painful, watery red eye, with photophobia and a history of trauma

What is seen on examination?

Conjunctival injection, a visible FB on the cornea and/or corneal abrasions staining with fluorescein

How is it managed?

The following steps need to be taken into account:

1. FB needs to be removed under the slit lamp with an 18 gauge needle (needle is used to flick FB out of eye)
2. Assess for a penetrating eye injury; look for iris defect, irregular pupil, soft eye
3. All high-speed injuries with metal FB need X-ray of the orbit
4. For corneal abrasions, and after removal of corneal FB, give chloramphenicol ointment qds for 5 days

PART III

SUBCONJUNCTIVAL HAEMORRHAGE

What is it?	Blood underneath the conjunctiva. Can involve a sector or the entire eye. Often painless
How is it caused?	Coughing, straining, hypertension, bleeding disorder, trauma, idiopathic
What should be obtained from the history?	The following information: 1. History of HTN (and check BP) 2. History of bleeding disorder 3. Medications: aspirin or warfarin 4. History of trauma
If traumatic, what must be done?	Full examination to rule out facial fracture/orbit injury
How is it managed?	Depends on the cause. Usually no treatment is required. Artificial tears if ocular irritation is present

BLEPHARITIS

What is it?	Inflammation of the lid margins
How does it present?	*Symptoms*: itching, burning, FB sensation, crusting around the lid margins early am *Signs*: crusty, red, thickened lid margins *Treatment*: lid scrub of lid margins (baby shampoo on a cotton bud) twice daily for 6 weeks If moderate, add occ. fusidic acid bd for 2 weeks If severe, refer to ophthalmologists for consideration of doxycycline oral treatment

DRY EYE SYNDROME

What causes it?

Unknown (idiopathic), connective tissue disease (rheumatoid arthritis, Sjögren's, SLE), drugs, post radiation, post laser

How does it present?

Symptoms: FB sensation, burning, reflex epiphora (watery eyes in wind, smoke, heat, prolonged use eg on computer)

Signs: low tear meniscus; increased tear break-up time (measured using fluorescein; time from a blink to the appearance of tear defect on the cornea)

Treatment: Viscotears®. If moderate–severe refer to ophthalmologist

GLAUCOMA

What types of glaucoma do you know of?

There are 2 types which are important to distinguish from each other:

1. Acute angle closure glaucoma (AACG)
2. Primary open angle glaucoma (POAG)

ACUTE ANGLE CLOSURE GLAUCOMA (AACG)

How does it present?

Painful red eye, nausea, vomiting, headache, blurred vision, halos around lights

What are the clinical findings?

Conjunctival injection, corneal oedema, fixed and mid-dilated pupil, high IOP

What is the treatment?

Refer to ophthalmologist ASAP.
Treatment includes:
1. Topical beta-blocker
2. Topical steroid
3. Carbonic anhydrase inhibitor (eg acetazolamide)
4. Pupil constrictor

Once corneal oedema settles, need **YAG laser peripheral iridotomy** to create alternative draining pathway for aqueous humor

PRIMARY OPEN ANGLE GLAUCOMA (POAG)

What are the risk factors?

Family history, black race, myopia, age, hypertension

How does it present?

Usually asymptomatic until the later stages, where patients may complain of visual field loss

What are the clinical findings?

The majority of patients will have raised IOP (>21 mmHg). The optic nerve has characteristic changes:
1. Thinning of the neuro-retinal rim
2. Disc haemorrhages
3. Notching
4. Cup-disc asymmetry
5. Enlarged cup-disc ratio

What are the investigations?

1. IOP measurement
2. Optic nerve examination
3. Visual field testing

What is the management?

Managed by ophthalmologists as a routine outpatient follow-up. The aim is to slow down the progression of the field defect by lowering the IOP. Most patients respond to **topical therapy**, but some may need surgery (trabeculoplasty), or laser trabeculoplasty.

Topical treatment includes beta-blockers, α_2-agonists, carbonic anhydrase inhibitors or prostaglandin agonists, which work by lowering the IOP

CATARACT

What is it?

Opacification of the lens

What are the causes?

Many:
1. Congenital
2. Age-related
3. Diabetes
4. Trauma
5. Inflammatory
6. Drug-induced (eg steroids)
7. Radiation
8. Hypocalcaemia
9. Myotonic dystrophy
10. Down's syndrome

How can they be remembered?

Mnemonic: **ABCDE**
Age-related
Bang (trauma, other injuries, including radiation)
Congenital, **C**alcium deficiency
Diabetes, **D**own's syndrome, **D**rugs (steroids)
Eye disease (glaucoma, uveitis)

What types do you know of?

The following:
1. Nuclear (central lens opacity)
2. Posterior subcapsular (opacities in the posterior aspect of the lens)
3. Cortical (radial opacities in the periphery)
4. Mixed

How do cataracts present?

Gradual deterioration in vision, glare around lights

PART III

What are the investigations?	Look for a cause, especially blood glucose. Complete ocular examination including dilated fundoscopy
How is it treated?	Consider surgical intervention if symptomatic. This is in the form of **phacoemulsification** and **lens implant**.

RETINAL DISORDERS

What causes these?	Localised disease, trauma, or as a manifestation of systemic diseases. They tend to be painless but of serious consequence to visual function (acuity, visual fields)

RETINAL DETACHMENT

How does it present?	**Floaters**, flashing lights, field loss, fall in visual acuity
What are the clinical findings?	Direct ophthalmoscopy: elevated retina, appears grey and balloons forward
What are the risk factors?	Myopia, past history of detachment or retinal tear, previous trauma or surgery
How is it managed?	Needs **urgent assessment** by an ophthalmologist, especially when the macula is still attached (acuity preserved)

CENTRAL RETINAL ARTERY OCCLUSION

What are the causes?	1. Embolus 2. Thrombus 3. Giant cell arteritis 4. Coagulopathies 5. Connective tissue diseases (SLE, PAN)

How does it present? — Unilateral, painless sudden loss of vision

What are the signs? — Relative afferent pupillary defect (RAPD). Direct ophthalmoscopy: pale retina with **cherry red spot** over the macula

What is RAPD? — Also known as Marcus–Gunn pupil. Using the swinging light test, light is shone into one eye, and then quickly switched to the other. This is repeated back and forth. Moderate RAPD: one pupil shows sustained constriction, followed by dilation to a greater size. Severe RAPD: one pupil shows an immediate dilation to a greater size. RAPD indicates pathology in the optic nerve or an extensive retinal lesion

What are the investigations? — **Blood investigations**:
1. ESR, autoantibody screen (giant cell arteritis/connective tissue disease screen)
2. Fasting glucose, lipid profile (diabetes/arteriopath/thrombus risk)
3. Clotting (coagulopathy screen)
Cardiac assessment: carotid Doppler, echo (?clot source)

How is it managed? — No single treatment has proved effective. Ocular massage and anterior chamber paracentesis (aqueous withdrawal from the anterior chamber)

CENTRAL RETINAL VEIN OCCLUSION

What are the causes?

1. Atherosclerosis
2. Hypertension
3. Glaucoma
4. Hypercoagulability
5. Drugs (eg OCP)
6. Vasculitis

How does it present?

Unilateral painless loss of vision

What are the signs?

Dilated tortuous veins. Retinal haemorrhages in all 4 quadrants of the retina

What are the investigations?

First, check BP to r/o HTN
Blood investigations:
1. Fasting glucose, lipid profile (diabetes/atherosclerosis screen)
2. Autoantibody screen, ESR (vasculitis/hypercoagulability screen)
Complete cardiovascular examination

What is the treatment?

Aspirin unless contraindicated
Refer to ophthalmologist for complete ocular examination including fundus fluorescein angiography (FFA)

VITREOUS HAEMORRHAGE

What are the causes?

1. Diabetic retinopathy
2. Ocular trauma
3. Retinal tear/detachment
4. Sickle cell disease
5. Retinal vein occlusion

How does it present?

Sudden-onset painless loss of vision. Black/red floaters

What are the findings?

Fundal view may be obscured by blood, with loss of the red reflex

What are the investigations?	Review of all systems in an aim to elucidate the cause Ocular exam by ophthalmologist. If there's no retinal view, perform a **B scan** (USS of the eye)
What is the treatment?	Depends on the aetiology. Advise patient on bedrest and **stop** aspirin or NSAID unless contraindicated

AGE-RELATED MACULAR DEGENERATION (ARMD)

What is the macula?	The yellow spot on the retina which represents the greatest concentration of cones, and is therefore the area of greatest visual acuity (syn. **macula lutea**)
What types of ARMD do you know of?	There are two types: **dry** (non-exudative) and **wet** (exudative)

DRY ARMD

How does it present?	**Gradual** distortion/loss of central vision
What are the signs?	Pigmentary changes over the macula with **macular drusen** (round, raised whitish lesions)
What are the investigations?	Important to distinguish from the wet type. Need ocular examination by ophthalmologist: FFA
How is it treated?	High-dose vitamin combination tablet (eg Ocuvite®) has been shown to reduce the risk of vision loss but only if they've never been smokers. Low vision aids may be of use in severe visual loss

WET ARMD

How does it present?	**Rapid**-onset loss of central vision. Distortion of straight lines

What are the signs?	Drusen with choroidal neovascular membrane (grey membrane underneath the retina). There may be subretinal haemorrhages
What are the risk factors?	Blue eyes, positive family history, smoking, age, hypertension
What are the investigations?	Assessment by an ophthalmologist as soon as possible for FFA
How is it treated?	Depending on the findings of the FFA. Options include laser photocoagulation, photodynamic therapy, ranibizumab or pegaptanib intravitreal injections (new anti-angiogenic factors)

RETINITIS PIGMENTOSA

What is it?	An inherited disorder, presenting with poor night vision and loss of peripheral field of vision
What is its mode of inheritance?	It can be autosomal dominant, autosomal recessive or X-linked recessive
What are the clinical findings?	Pigment clumps in peripheral retina (**'bone spicules'**)
How is it managed?	Assessment and genetic counselling at a specialist centre

TOXOPLASMOSIS

How does it present?	With blurred vision and floaters. It is painless
What are the clinical findings?	New whitish retinal lesion. There may be an old pigmented retinal scar. Inflammatory cells may be present in the anterior chamber

What are the investigations?	Complete ocular examination by ophthalmologist Anti-toxoplasmosis antibody titre Consider HIV test if high-risk patient
What is the treatment?	Triple therapy with pyrimethamine, sulfadiazine and folinic acid

DIABETIC RETINOPATHY

How does it present?	In 4 main different forms: 1. **Maculopathy**: macula is thickened due to oedema and hard exudates may be present 2. **Background DR** (mild non-proliferative DR): dot-blot haemorrhages, microaneurysms and hard exudates 3. **Non-proliferative DR** (moderate and severe DR): same findings of background DR plus cotton wool spots (ischaemic areas of retina) and venous beading 4. **Proliferative DR**: new vessels are present at the optic disc (new vessels at disc, NVD) or elsewhere in the retina (new vessels elsewhere, NVE) or in the iris (rubeosis)
What are the risk factors?	Hypertension, duration of diabetes, poor glycaemic control, hyperlipidaemia, presence of diabetic nephropathy
How is it investigated?	All diabetics need annual dilated fundal check; if retinopathy is present then review needs to be more frequent depending on the severity of disease. In case of maculopathy they will need FFA. Check BP and screen for hyperlipidaemia

PART III

What is the treatment?	Non-ischaemic maculopathy requires laser surrounding the macula (grid) Proliferative DR requires pan retinal photocoagulation (PRP)

HYPERTENSIVE RETINOPATHY

How is this classified?	As follows:	
	Grade 1	Silver wiring (tortuous vessels with shiny walls)
	Grade 2	A-V nipping (narrowing at artery and vein cross-over)
	Grade 3	Flame haemorrhages and cotton wool spots
	Grade 4	Swelling of optic disc (previously called papilloedema)
What is the management?	Pharmacological control of BP. Grade 4 is a medical emergency as blindness can ensue	

THE EYE IN SYSTEMIC DISEASE

What eye signs may be found in the following systemic illnesses?

Graves' disease?	1. Proptosis 2. Lid retraction and lid lag 3. Conjunctival chemosis 4. Dry cornea 5. Diplopia due to extraocular muscle infiltration 6. Optic nerve atrophy
Sarcoidosis?	1. Iris nodules 2. Anterior uveitis 3. Lacrimal gland infiltration causing dry eyes 4. Posterior uveitis

Wilson's disease?	Kayser–Fleischer rings (copper deposition in cornea)
Homocystinuria?	1. Lens dislocation (downward) 2. Cataract
Marfan's syndrome?	1. Lens dislocation (upward) 2. Myopia 3. Retinal tears and detachment
AIDS?	Susceptible to opportunistic infections: 1. Molluscum contagiosum 2. HZO 3. Bacterial and fungal keratitis 4. CMV retinitis 5. Toxoplasmosis Also prone to: 1. HIV retinopathy 2. Kaposi sarcoma of the lids
What is temporal arteritis?	A form of giant cell arteritis (a vasculitis)
What is its claim to fame?	It is an ophthalmological emergency!
How does it present?	With the following symptoms: 1. **Sudden-onset visual loss**, usually unilateral 2. Temple pain/headache 3. Jaw claudication (pain on chewing) 4. May have history of **polymyalgia rheumatica**
What are the signs?	The following: 1. Poor visual acuity (including **blindness**) 2. Relative afferent papillary defect 3. Absent temporal artery pulsation in a thickened, ropy-feeling temporal artery 4. Pale optic disc
What are the investigations?	An **urgent** ESR (will be raised), and a temporal artery biopsy

PART III

227

What should be done if the ESR comes back as high?

Start treatment **immediately** to prevent blindness. Do this *before* even considering biopsy!

What *is* the treatment?

High-dose oral steroids

Why does temporal arteritis cause visual disturbance/blindness?

The temporal artery (a branch of the external carotid a.) anastomoses with the ophthalmic artery (a branch of the internal carotid a.), which supplies the eye

SOCIAL IMPLICATIONS

What are the visual requirements for driving in the UK?

The DVLA requirements include rules on visual acuity, fields, colour blindness and diplopia

Their requirement for visual acuity is 'to read in good light (with the aid of glasses or contact lenses if worn) a registration mark fixed to a motor vehicle and containing letters and figures 79 millimetres high and 50 millimetres wide (ie post 1.9.2001 font) at a distance of 20 metres, or at a distance of 20.5 metres where the characters are 79 millimetres high and 57 millimetres wide (i.e. pre 1.9.2001 font). If unable to meet this standard, the driver must not drive and the licence must be refused or revoked.'

(Also: http://www.dvla.gov.uk/media/pdf/medical/aagv1.pdf)

CHAPTER 10: PLASTIC SURGERY

TRAUMA IN PLASTIC SURGERY

What specific points are important in the plastics history?

1. **Timing**: what time did the injury occur?
2. **Where**: was it in a clean or dirty environment? Was it at work or at home?
3. **How**: exactly what was the mechanism, eg crush or cut; if crushed, how long for, what caused the crush, how was the part released?
4. **Foreign body**: is there the possibility of a foreign body in the wound?
5. **Treatment so far**: what treatment has been administered so far and when?
6. **PMHx**: include history of prior surgery/injury to the affected area. Assess co-morbidity
7. **DHx**: current medications, allergies

UPPER LIMB EXAMINATION

How is examination of the upper limb approached?

Look, feel, move. Try to cause as little pain to the patient as possible

What are the important points in looking?

1. **Obvious wounds**: observe all the skin of the limb: there may be distracting injuries in one area masking a severe injury in another

Assess the wound: note the following:

i. Dirty or clean?

ii. Neat cut or crushed?

iii. Adequate skin coverage for closure?

iv. Degloving (skin and fascia) or avulsion (deeper tissues) injury?

v. Evidence of infection?

2. **Resting position**: may be obvious with the patient clutching a painful area, or more subtle such as a break in the normal cascade of the fingers suggesting flexor tendon injury

3. **Circulation**: verify that the patient does not have compromised circulation to a distal part as a result of injury. Assess skin colour, capillary refill time, pulses

4. **Oedema**: swelling over digits or joints often points to an underlying bony injury

What adjuncts can be used to assess circulation?

Doppler ultrasound can be used. Allen test may be useful

What must be done if there is a possibility of circulation compromise?

The patient must be assessed for urgent exploration in operating theatre

What should be felt for?

1. Skin temperature
2. Feel over bones and joints for evidence of swelling and pain which may indicate an underlying bony injury
3. Find evidence of nerve damage by testing sensation (described later)

What movements should be checked?

Passive and active motion, and motion against force

What are the flexor tendons of the hand?	Flexor digitorum superficialis (FDS) and flexor digitorum profundus (FDP)
How is FDS tested?	**Function**: FDS flexes the proximal interphalangeal joint (PIPJ) and joints proximal to that **Test**: stabilise the metacarpophalangeal joint (MCPJ) and ask the patient to bend their finger. FDP contributes to the flexion, as can be seen by movement at the DIPJ. This can be eliminated in the ulnar three digits, to which FDP tendons have a common muscle belly. Therefore, by holding the other two digits in extension, a pure FDS movement can be elicited in the examined finger
And FDP?	**Function**: FDP flexes the DIPJ and joints proximal to that **Test**: stabilise the PIPJ and ask the patient to bend the end of the finger
How are the hand extensors tested?	Ask the patient to extend all digits, paying particular attention to specific joints involved in injury
What thumb movements must be examined?	Flexion, extension, abductor, adductor and opposition
How can flexor tendon injury be classified?	Into zones which are relevant to management planning and outcome; these should be documented in the clerking (See Table 10.1)

Table 10.1

Zone	Anatomical region
I	FDP alone distal to FDS insertion
II	From proximal end of zone I to proximal end of fibro-osseous tunnel
III	Area in palm where flexor tendons are free of any fibrous pulleys
IV	Carpal canal area
V	Proximal end of carpal tunnel to the musculo-tendinous junction

What about extensor injury?

Also into zones: I–IX. Similar to the flexor tendon classification, zone I is the most distal and zone IX is proximal forearm injuries. The zone of injury is again relevant to planning of repair

Give an example of a Zone I extensor injury

Mallet finger, which can be managed conservatively with a mallet splint, which holds the DIPJ in extension. It is worn for 6 weeks allowing non-surgical healing

How are the digital nerves examined?

With 2-point discrimination on the ulnar and radial orders of each digit. This can be done using a paperclip

MEDIAN NERVE

What are the branches of the median nerve in the hand?

The median nerve divides into 2 in the palm, the lateral portion supplying the **thenar muscles** and lateral sensation, and the medial portion supplying the **lumbricals** and medial sensation

The **palmar branch** arises at the lower forearm and pierces the **carpal ligament**. It then divides into lateral and medial branches in the hand, which supply sensation to the skin over the base of the thumb and the palm respectively

What are the thenar muscles?

Mnemonic: **LOAF**
Lateral 2 lumbricals
Opponens pollicis
Abductor pollicis brevis
Flexor pollicis longus

How is it examined?

Sensory: test sensation to the lateral three and a half digits (ie thumb, index, middle and lateral half of ring with palm facing upwards)
Motor: ask the patient to put their palm facing up and point their thumb in the air, tell them to keep it in that position whilst you try and push it down towards their palm

ULNAR NERVE

What are the branches of the ulnar nerve in the hand?

The ulnar nerve divides into a deep motor and superficial sensory branch just beyond the **pisiform bone**. Its *sensory supply* is to the medial one and a half digits. Its *motor supply* is to the intrinsic muscles of the hand (medial three lumbricals and the interossei) and **adductor pollicis** Isolated sensory loss is possible with certain injuries

How is it examined?

Sensory: test sensation to the medial one and a half digits (ie little finger and medial half of the ring with the palm facing upwards)

PART III

Motor: ask the patient to hold a piece of paper between thumb and radial side of index finger whilst you try and pull it away using your thumb and index finger. If adductor pollicis is weak then compensation by **flexor pollicis longus** will lead to an excessively flexed posture of the thumb IPJ. (**Froment's sign**)

RADIAL NERVE

What are the branches of the radial nerve in the hand?

There are no major branches in the hand

What does it supply?

Its *sensory supply* is to the extensor surface (dorsum) of the hand and forearm. Its *motor supply* is to the hand extensors

How is it tested?

Sensory: test sensation over the dorsum of the 1st web space
Motor: ask patient to hold his hand out flat, palm down. Ask him to hold it straight whilst you push down on the fingers

NERVE INJURY

What types of peripheral nerve injury are there?

Neuropraxia, axonotmesis and neurotmesis.

What is neuropraxia?

Temporary conduction block from modest compression or traction. All components of the nerve remain intact

What is axonotmesis?

Loss of axonal continuity, but surrounding connective tissue sheath remains intact
Regeneration from proximal nerve advances at 1 mm/day

How may axonotmesis be detected clinically?

With **Tinel's sign**: tapping over site of injury causes paraesthesia distally

What is neurotmesis?

Loss of continuity of axon and complete disruption of connective tissue sheath. Likely to form **neuroma**

What are the indications for a nerve repair?

In a sharp **transection injury**, a repair should be carried out straight away
If the injury is **blunt**, it may be necessary to observe the deficit and use **EMG testing** in order to define what type of injury has been sustained before making a management decision

How is a nerve repair performed?

It can be a **primary repair** or a **nerve graft**. Small sutures are used (8–0 to 10–0 monofilament) and the repair is tension-free. A splint is worn post operatively for 3 weeks allowing only intermittent movement in a protected range

What is the outcome of nerve repair?

In patients who have had a digital nerve repair, two-thirds have a good sensory recovery (return of pain and touch sensation)

TENDON INJURY

What surrounds a tendon?

Tendon is either surrounded by paratenon or tendon sheath

What is the paratenon?

Paratenon exists where the tendon is not subjected to mechanical stress. It consists of connective tissue and synovial cells and bathes the tendon in a fluid environment. Within it is **epitenon** containing vascular, lymphatic and nerve supply in a loose connective tissue

What is the tendon sheath?

This exists in areas of mechanical stress. It is made up of two layers. The outer **fibrotic layer** is continuous with annular and cruciate pulleys. The inner layer is a **synovial sheath**

What are pulleys?

Thickenings of the flexor tendon sheath that holds the tendon in place over joints and phalanges. They prevent bowstringing of the tendon, ie migration in a volar direction. The most crucial are the A2 and A4 pulleys (see Table 10.2)

Table 10.2

Pulley	Position
A1	Just proximal to the MCPJ
A2	Over the proximal phalanx
A3	Over the PIPJ
A4	Over the middle phalanx
A5	Over the DIPJ

What is the pre-op management of an open tendon injury?

1. Give analgesia
2. Consider tetanus
3. Clean and irrigate the wound as soon as possible under local anaesthesia
4. Dress with non-adherent sterile material
5. Apply splint to immobilise
6. Elevate
7. Consider antibiotics, especially if the patient has waited or will wait more than 6 hours for repair
8. Prepare the patient for theatre (consent, anaesthetic review, investigations as needed)

When is a tendon injury repaired?

As soon as possible. A primary repair is within 12 hours; delayed primary is within 10–14 days; secondary is within 2–4 weeks; and late repair after 4 weeks

Some reasons or delay are:

1. Other significant injury requiring prompt attention
2. Grossly contaminated wound
3. Co-morbidity preventing anaesthesia

What are the indications for repair?

Tendon injury associated with a clean wound, and replantation

What does repair involve?

It is usually done under general anaesthetic. There are many types of tendon repair but Kessler repair is often used. Following repair, splintage is applied and the limb is elevated. Antibiotics are usually given

What are the complications of tendon repair?

Early: haematoma, infection, rupture of tendon repair or pulley, poor wound healing, poor tendon glide within its sheath

Later: late tendon rupture, adhesions and joint contractures, scar problems

What is the post-op management following tendon repair?

Can range from immobilisation to early controlled **following tendon** motion. The latter is generally instituted and must be arranged with the hand physiotherapist as an out-patient programme. Other considerations are antibiotic cover, elevation and organising follow-up

REPLANT

What is a replant?

The reattaching of an amputated part of the body. The most common is digital replant

PART III

How should an amputated part be stored in transit?	**Protected** within a cold environment. For example, a digit can be wrapped in gauze and placed in a sealed waterproof bag. This is then put in a bag of ice *It is important that the amputated part is not put directly in to contact with ice or it will become macerated!*
What can be replanted?	Any body part brought in should be considered by a senior surgeon
What factors affect viability?	These include: 1. Level of amputation 2. Quality of the amputation, ie clean cut better than crush 3. Part amputated, eg a dominant thumb is more important than a non-dominant little finger 4. Co-morbidity 5. Attitude of the patient
What is ischaemia time?	The time measured from **devascularisation** (time of injury) to **revascularisation** (re-establishment of arterial flow). Replant is not usually recommended if this is >6 hours for injury proximal to the wrist, or > 16 hours for digital amputation
What is the operative sequence of replanting?	Bone, artery, flexor tendon, extensor tendon, vein
What is important in post-op?	Hydration and analgesia. Adjuncts such as dextran, chlorpromazine, aspirin and heparin may be used to improve survival of the replanted part

OTHER HAND INJURIES

What are the features of a nail bed injury?	More common in men. Occurs with a history of crush injury to the finger tip, such as trapping it in a car door

What is a subungual haematoma?

A haematoma under the nail. It indicates laceration to the nail bed. Consider underlying fracture of the distal phalanx (which technically makes it a compound fracture)

What is the management of nail bed injury?

1. Remove nail under digital ring block
2. Repair nail bed either with primary closure or with grafting if the laceration is messy
3. Replace nail or a piece of material of similar shape after the repair in order to keep the **nail fold** open

How fast does new nail grow?

At a rate of 1 mm/day

What other common hand injuries occur?

Animal and human bites are often to the hand

What is a 'fight bite'?

A human bite wound sustained as the patient's fist hits the mouth of his opponent (usually on a Saturday night!)

What is its danger?

Can lead to MCP joint space infection which requires surgical washout and drainage, and antibiotic therapy

What must be remembered?

When animal or human bites are deep enough that the base of the wound cannot be seen, they require laying open for irrigation and debridement in addition to antibiotic therapy in order to prevent abscess formation

What is suppurative tenosynovitis?

Suppurative infection in the flexor tendon sheath, usually following a puncture wound, which has the potential to spread proximally

PART III

What are the findings?	The clinical features are: 1. Semiflexed posture 2. Fusiform swelling 3. Tenderness over the flexor tendon 4. Pain with passive motion of tendon
What is the outcome?	Severe impairment of function if not treated surgically with a flexor sheath wash-out

BURNS

CLINICAL ANATOMY

What are the layers of the skin?	The skin consists of two main layers: the epidermis and dermis
What are the properties of the epidermis?	It is essentially **avascular.** Its function is **cornification**, which is creation of a tough layer of dead cells
How thick is it?	It is 0.04–1.6 mm thick depending on the site (thicker on the palms and soles, thinner on the eyelids)
What cells constitute the epidermis?	Epidermis contains four types of cells: keratinocyte, melanocyte, Langerhan's cell and Merkel cell
What are the properties of the dermis?	It contains the vascular bed of the skin and its function is **temperature regulation**. It also contains nerves and glandular elements of the skin
How thick is it?	It is 15–40 times thicker than the epidermis. It can be divided into two layers: the **superficial papillary layer** and the **deep reticular layer**

CLINICAL CONSIDERATIONS

What is a burn?

Damage to the skin resulting from an external insult which can lead to a local and systemic reaction

What are the zones of a burn?

Three zones in all:
Zone of coagulation: the burn epicentre
Zone of ischaemia or stasis: the area peripheral or deep to the burn which is initially viable but has the potential to become devitalised if fluid resuscitation is insufficient
Zone of hyperaemia: the outermost area where there is vasodilatation in response to the injury but the tissue remains viable

What are the physiological effects of a burn?

Tissue damage leads to release of tissue mediators (serotonin, prostaglandin, complement, histamine, platelet products) which cause capillary leak into the interstitial space
→ The leak progresses until the interstitium is iso-osmotic with the intravascular compartment
→ This **third-spacing** is made worse by structural damage from the irreversible denaturing of collagen, which increases the negative pressure of the third space

What are the clinical effects?

Always keep the following in mind:
• Immediate/ life-threatening effects are inhalation injury and uncompensated fluid losses. Patients with 15–20% total body surface area (TBSA) burns will be shocked, the maximal effects being 6–12 hours post burn

- The patient may develop a systemic inflammatory response syndrome (SIRS)
- Burns are extremely painful
- Circumferential burns can cause compartment syndrome

A patient is referred with a burn injury; what information do you need prior to their arrival?

The following:

The patient: personal details, significant co-morbidity, associated injuries, relevant drug/alcohol history

The burn: type (thermal, chemical, electrical); percentage and depth; timing; anatomical areas affected with associated information (eg genital burn: has the patient been catheterised?)

Treatment given: airway management/anaesthetic review; fluids administered; drugs administered; dressings applied; management of associated injuries

The patient arrives in the department; what is the order of assessment?

ABCs! When stabilised continue on to secondary survey and full history

How do you recognise airway compromise in a burns patient?

May be obvious with stridor and dyspnoea, or may be more subtle

What are the risk factors?

Risk factors are:
1. History of unconsciousness
2. History of an enclosed space
3. Singed nasal hairs
4. Soot around the airway on examination
5. Production of carbonaceous sputum

If there is a question over airway compromise, ask for an anaesthetic assessment and perform blood gas analysis and a plain chest radiograph

How is circulation supported in a burns patient?

Gain large-bore intravenous access and ensure adequate hydration with the rapid initiation of fluids. Try and place cannulae on unburnt tissue as it will be easier to secure and less likely to become displaced by developing oedema

How much fluid should be given?

Parkland Formula is commonly used for adult burns:
3–4 ml/kg per %TBSA burn of Hartman's solution over 24 hours
The first half is given in the first 8 hours post burn, and the second half given over the remaining 16 hours
It is important to include in your calculations what fluid has already been given at the referring centre

What analgesia can be used?

Burns can be very painful: use opiates

What investigations should be done?

Use common sense depending on severity of burn.
Bedside investigations:
1. ECG
2. Urine dip-stick
3. Urine myoglobin
Blood investigations:
1. GXM
2. ABG
3. Carbon monoxide levels
Imaging: chest radiograph to r/o pulmonary insult
Other:
1. Wound swabs for microbiology
2. Nasopharyngoscopy may be required to assess upper airway for oedema

What should be considered?

Urinary catheter, central venous catheterisation and nasogastric tube

| **How are the wounds managed?** | They must be assessed and documented and then cleaned, de-roofed and dressed |
| **How is a burn wound classified?** | See Table 10.3 |

Table 10.3

Classification	Description
Superficial	Epidermal damage. No blister, blanches, erythematous, painful. Conservative management
Partial thickness (PTB) (superficial dermal)	Papillary dermal elements damaged. Blisters, blanches, painful. Conservative management
Partial thickness (deep dermal)	Deep dermal damage. No blistering, weak blanching, usually painful, may require surgical management
Full thickness (FTB)	Damage to and beyond subcutaneous layer. Non-blanching, leathery, not painful. Surgical management

| **How is percentage burn estimated?** | Using a **Lund and Browder chart** is the most accurate way of estimating and documenting percentage burn (see Figure 10.1)
The **rule of 9s** can also be used: head 9%, arms 9% each, legs 18% each, trunk 18% front, 18% back, perineum 1%. The patient's palm can be used as a rough measure of 1% TBSA
In children the proportional dimensions of the body are different, therefore the Lund and Browder chart is different for children |

Figure 10.1

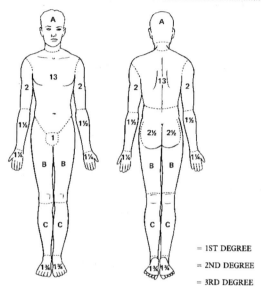

BURN SHEET

Name .... AGE .... NUMBER ....

BURN RECORD. AGES 7 TO ADULT.   DATE OF OBSERVATION ....

= 1ST DEGREE
= 2ND DEGREE
= 3RD DEGREE

RELATIVE PERCENTAGES OF AREAS AFFECTED BY GROWTH

AREA	AGE 10	15	ADULT
A ½ OF HEAD	5½	4½	3½
B ½ OF ONE THIGH	4¼	4½	4¾
C ½ OF ONE LEG	3	3¼	3½

% BURN BY AREAS

PROBABLE 3RD° BURN { HEAD ... NECK ... BODY ... UP. ARM ... FOREARM ... HANDS .... GENITALS ..... BUTTOCKS ..... THIGHS ..... LEGS ...... FEET ......

TOTAL BURN { HEAD ... NECK ... BODY ... UP. ARM .... FOREARM ... HANDS .... GENITALS ..... BUTTOCKS ..... THIGHS ..... LEGS ...... FEET ......

Who needs surgery?

1. FTB > 1 cm in diameter: debridement and grafting
2. Burn causing thoracic constriction: escharotomy
3. Contaminated, dirty burn: formal debridement
4. Other circumferential burns causing compartment syndrome (see Chapter 5, 'Compartment syndrome')

What is an electrical burn?

Damage sustained when an electrical current passes through the body from an entry point to an exit point, disrupting tissues and structures through which it passes

How is a patient with an electrical burn assessed?

As always, ABCs, then secondary survey
History: voltage, type of current (alternating or direct), time in contact, timing of incident, part of body in contact, loss of consciousness, associated injuries
Examination: entry and exit points, as part of full physical examination, look for associated injuries and specific effects such as cardiac arrhythmias and compartment syndrome. Check inside the **mouth** as this is an area of **low resistance**

What are the possible outcomes of an electrical burn?

The following:
1. Damage to any tissues in the path of the current (skin, muscle, organs, bone)
2. Arrhythmias are common
3. The effects of muscle breakdown (eg myoglobinuria and resultant renal failure)

So what investigations should be done?

Blood investigations:
1. FBC
2. U&E: may be altered in renal failure
3. LFT: r/o liver damage

Bedside investigations:
1. ECG to look for arrhythmias
2. Urine myoglobin

Radiology: obtain radiographs if bony injury/ dislocation is suspected (remember to look for posterior shoulder dislocation)

Other: consider cardiac monitoring, especially if arrhythmias seen on ECG

What is the management of an electrical burn?

Depends on the type and severity of burn; ranges from wound dressing and observant cardiac monitoring to amputation of limbs

What is a chemical burn?

The process occurring when a chemical comes into contact with the skin causing damage through the skin layers mainly as a result of the chemical reaction, with the potential to cause systemic effects

What types of chemical burn are there?

1. Alkaline
2. Acid
3. Corrosive
4. Oxidising and reducing agents
5. Vesicants
6. Protoplasmic poison (eg hydrofluoric acid)

What is a vesicant?

A highly reactive chemical that reacts with proteins, DNA and other cellular components, resulting in immediate cellular changes. Used in chemical warfare, eg sulphur mustard, lewisite

PART III

What are the important aspects of the history?

Find out what caused the burn, its concentration or strength, time of exposure, period of exposure and first aid so far administered

What is the management of a chemical burn?

1. Early irrigation with water; acid is more easily neutralised than alkali, requiring 2–3 hours of irrigation compared to over 12 hours required for alkali
2. Remove clothing and visible particles from the wound

Burning will not stop until the agent is neutralised. Once irrigation is complete, the wound should be reassessed

What is hydrofluoric acid?

An inorganic acid used mainly in industry which can cause local and systemic toxicity from cutaneous exposure and inhalation. Cutaneous exposure causes delayed-onset intense pain and tissue destruction. Hydrofluoric acid has a predilection for **subungual tissue**

What is the management of exposure to hydrofluoric acid?

1. Irrigation with water for 15–30 minutes
2. If pain continues then the acid is still burning the skin, detoxify with calcium: remove all blisters then apply topical calcium gluconate gel and secure it in place with an occlusive latex cover, eg a glove. If the burn is deep the the gel will not penetrate far enough. In these cases infiltrative calcium therapy should be used (10% calcium gluconate)

3. Monitor for systemic effects of hydrofluoric acid toxicity such as cardiac dysrhythmia and electrolyte imbalance. Hydrofluoric acid binds with magnesium and calcium with a strong affinity

WOUND HEALING AND SCARRING

What is a problem wound?

Problem wounds are those that have failed to heal up spontaneously by primary or secondary intention

What are the causes?

Can be classified into wound factors or patient factors:

Wound factors:
1. Vascular insufficiency
2. Infected wound
3. Cavity wound
4. Fistula
5. Mechanical stress from pressure or trauma

Patient factors:
1. Diabetes
2. Sepsis
3. Malignant disease
4. Vasculitis
5. Poor nutrition
6. Obesity

How can these also be remembered?

Mnemonic: **VITAMINS A, B, C, D, E**

Vitamin deficiency
Infection (local and generalised)
Technique
Arterial supply (especially vascular disease or trauma)
Malnutrition
Icterus (2ry to hepatobiliary disease, haemolysis or uraemia)
Necrotic tissue
Sugar (diabetes mellitus)

PART III

Anaemia, **A**ge
Blood clot (haematoma formation)
Cancer (local or distant)
Drugs (cytotoxic agents and steroids)
Edge tension (esp. in **obesity**)

What are the non-operative management options?

Conservative: address the environment (eg pressure sore prevention) and minimise patient factors as far as possible (eg prevention of malnutrition)
Medical: the following:
1. Topical antimicrobials
2. Systemic antibiotics
3. Irrigation
4. Specialist dressings
5. Hyperbaric oxygen can be considered

The above should be done as part of a multidisciplinary team

What is a VAC dressing?

A specialist vacuum-assisted dressing. It operates by maintaining a sub-atmospheric pressure at the surface of the wound using a vacuum pump

How does it work?

It helps restore blood flow and granulation tissue to the wound. There are intermittent and constant pressure settings and the dressing is changed every 2–3 days

What are the surgical options?

Debridement: surgical removal of devitalised, infected or necrotic tissue or fibrin from the surface of a wound until healthy bleeding tissue is exposed

How does debridement work?

It converts a chronic wound into an acute 'fresh' wound giving it a new opportunity to granulate or act as the recipient bed for a graft

What are problem scars?

Scars that heal abnormally. There are two types: hypertrophic and keloid.

What is a hypertrophic scar?

A red, raised and sometimes itchy scar that does *not* extend over normal tissue

What is the natural history?

It has the potential to grow for 3–6 months and then it has the potential to regress. It can take up to 2 years to reach maturity, and when it does its appearance is elevated and rope-like

What is a keloid scar?

An abnormal scar that extends into normal tissue
It can be classified as minor or major

What is the natural history?

Minor keloid: raised and itchy, extending into normal tissue. It may develop up to 1 year after the initial injury and it does not have the potential to regress
Major keloid: large raised scar which extends over normal tissue. It may be painful as well as itchy and can continue to spread for years

What are the risk factors for keloid scarring?

The following:
1. Young age
2. Pre-existing keloid
3. Dark-skinned races: commonest in black skin, followed by lighter skin (Asian, American Indian), followed by white skin
4. Location: it commonly affects the presternal area, deltoid area and earlobes

PART III

What is the management of keloid scars?

They do not respond to surgical excision as the keloid usually re-forms with the new scar. If a keloid *is* excised, it should be done **intra-lesionally** (keloid excised leaving a rim of scar tissue). Medical treatments are injection with triamcinolone or silicone gel (these should be given after excision as well, if performed)

What are the methods of wound closure and coverage used by plastic surgeons?

Direct closure, skin grafts and flaps

How can wounds be aesthetically improved?

By the following methods:
1. Meticulous direct closure technique
2. Siting the wound, where possible, along the natural lines of the skin
3. Specific techniques such as Z-plasty can be utilised to improve wounds that have healed in contracture
4. Non-linear incisions are used to prevent scar contracture primarily

SKIN GRAFTING

What types of skin graft are there?

Split thickness skin graft (SSG), full thickness skin graft (FTSG)

What are the indications for skin grafting?

Coverage of wounds that cannot be closed primarily due to skin loss, eg traumatic wound, burn wound, wound following tumour resection
Other indications are hair restoration, nipple-areola reconstruction and vitiligo

What are the pre-requisites for skin grafting?

In order for the graft to survive, the wound bed must have certain qualities: it must be vascular and free of infection or malignant disease

What are the contraindications for skin grafting?

Relative contraindications are those that give a less than optimal wound bed:
1. Previous irradiation
2. Vascular insufficiency
3. Wound abnormality
4. Bleeding abnormality

What is a split skin graft?

A graft harvested from the epidermis measuring 0.30–0.45 mm. It is above the level of the skin appendages so that hair follicles and sweat glands are not included in the graft

What different types do you know of?

Sheet graft: gives a uniform appearance to the healed wound
Perforated sheet graft: allows the escape of serous fluid
Meshed graft: can expand like a garden trellis and has a more comfortable fit on wound beds with irregular topography, but the meshed appearance is visible after wound healing

Where is a split skin graft taken from?

Anywhere on the body although the most used sites are the thigh, trunk and buttocks as they are easier to harvest from and relatively discreet

What qualities should the donor site possess?

It should provide an area of skin free of infection or carbuncles, that can be flattened. It should be shaved if it is hairy

What should patients be warned of?

The donor site remains scarred and discoloured when healed

PART III

What anaesthetic should be used to harvest the graft?

Local or general anaesthetic. Local anaesthetic can either be topical or infiltrated. If topical, the anaesthetic cream is spread liberally over the marked donor site and sealed on using a waterproof covering and tape. It should be left for at least an hour

How is the graft harvested?

Either freehand using a **harvesting knife** or (more commonly) an electrically powered hand-held **dermatome**

The surface must be moist, sterile and flattened and the graft taken should be slightly larger than the recipient site

Once the graft has been taken the wound is covered with a sterile dressing such as Kaltostat® and local anaesthetic is applied

How is it grafted?

By the following steps:

1. Prepare wound by removal of devitalised tissue and ensuring haemostasis
2. Prepare graft (it may be perforated or meshed) and placed on the donor site, carefully moulding it to the wound
3. Fix graft in place: it can be sutured (interrupted undyed vicryl) or glued; it can also be left unfixed
4. Apply non-adherent dressing and splint if necessary. The aim of the dressing and the splintage is to maintain a sterile environment and protect the graft from any movement or shearing force

What is a full thickness skin graft?

A graft that includes epidermis and dermis

How does it differ from a split skin graft clinically?

1. Less prone to contracture
2. Can match the surrounding skin better in texture and colour
3. Thick enough to maintain a uniform contour where an SSG would leave a concave defect. It therefore has a better aesthetic appearance
4. It includes adnexal structures including hair follicles

How does it differ from a split skin graft physiologically?

An SSG heals by epithelial migration whereas a FTSG is thought to survive initially by serum imbibition and then by revascularisation

When is a FTSG used instead of a SSG?

1. Sites where aesthetic result is important, eg the face
2. Sites where graft contracture would be problematic
3. Small recipient site

What donor site should be used for a FTSG?

1. A site where the skin is a similar colour and quality to the recipient area. For example a graft to the face should be taken from the 'blush zone' which is the area above the shoulders
2. The site should be in an area where the skin is mobile enough to allow direct closure and ideally in an area where the scar will be discreet

PART III

How is it grafted?

1. A template is made of the recipient area; this is marked and excised from the donor area
2. Subcutaneous fat is removed from the graft with sharp curved scissors to improve graft 'take'
3. The graft is secured using undyed vicryl (interrupted) in a fashion that there is no tension or blanching
4. A tie-over dressing or a regular non-adherent dressing with gentle pressure can be used

What is a tie-over dressing?

A pressure dressing which is tied down over the graft using sutures placed **radially** around the graft. It helps reduce the risk of seroma and haematoma formation and prevents any shearing force on the graft. It is usually left in place for 1–2 weeks

What leads to graft failure?

1. Inadequate bed: for example, a graft on exposed tendon (avascular) will be less likely to survive than a graft on paratenon which in turn will be less likely to survive than a graft on granulation tissue
2. Infection, especially with *Streptococcus pyogenes*
3. Mechanical stress, especially shearing
4. Haematoma
5. Seroma
6. Patient co-morbidity

FLAPS

What is a flap?

Another method for wound coverage or providing bulk. It is a graft with an intrinsic blood supply

How are flaps classified?

Based on one the following:
1. **Tissues which constitute the flap**: skin, fasciocutaneous, muscle, myocutaneous, osteomyocutaneous
2. **Blood supply**: random pattern or axial
3. **Distance of transposition**: local or distant

What types of local flaps are there?

Transposition flap: the flap moves laterally to fill a primary defect
Rotation flap: the flap is rotated into the defect
Advancement flap: the flap is advanced into the defect, eg a V-Y flap
These are all **random pattern flaps**: they rely on the random pattern of blood supply from the **subdermal plexus**. The flap length:width ratio is limited to 2:1 to ensure that the distal flap is adequately vascularised

What is a distant flap?

A flap of tissue transferred from one site of the body to another

What types of distant flaps are there?

A distant flap is either attached to a blood supply (**pedicle flap**) or disconnected from its original blood supply and reconnected by vascular anastomosis to suitable vessels in the recipient area (**free flap**)
These flaps are **axial flaps** based on specific vascular territories allowing a greater length:width ratio

PART III

What is delay?

This is surgically outlining the flap a few weeks prior to its transfer in order to improve its blood supply by giving it some 'safe time' do develop a more unidirectional supply

When is a flap used rather than a graft?

1. Coverage of an avascular wound bed
2. Coverage of a wound that has previously failed to take a graft
3. Coverage of a large area
4. Coverage of an area where bulk, sensation, cosmesis and lack of contracture is important
5. To provide bulk for aesthetic reasons (eg latissimus dorsi flap for breast reconstruction)

What should be considered pre-op when planning a flap?

Full history and examination should reveal previous incisions, muscle wasting, vascular supply and co-morbidity. Specific questions to be asked are:

1. Have swabs of the wound been performed for infecting/colonising bacteria?
2. Does vascular status need further investigation?
3. What surgical procedures have been performed so far?
4. Has there been any radiation therapy to this area?

What investigations should be done?

Special investigations may be required such as selective angiography, Doppler ultrasound studies and magnetic resonance angiography

What are the important aspects of early post-op management?

1. Regular flap monitoring as signs of ischaemia must be acted on promptly
2. Protect flap against pressure and elevated if possible

3. The patient should be kept well hydrated aiming initially for a urine output of 1 ml/kg per hour
4. Some surgeons use antibiotics and anticoagulants post operatively

How is the flap monitored?

Clinical observation: skin colour, tissue turgor, temperature and capillary refill time
Investigations: fluorescein, transcutaneous oxygen and Doppler ultrasound
Muscular flaps are less easy to monitor clinically but can be tested for muscle twitch with a gentle pinch

What are the complications of a flap?

Early complications:
1. Arterial insufficiency
2. Venous engorgement
3. Haemorrhage
Later complications:
1. Seroma
2. Haematoma
3. Infection
4. Superficial skin necrosis
5. Partial or complete loss of flap
6. Inadequate defect coverage
7. Donor site problems

What is the management of flap arterial insufficiency?

The flap is cold and pale with a slow capillary refill time (CRT): *this is an emergency*
1. Inform the operating surgeon
2. Prep patient for return to theatre
3. In the meantime keep the flap warm and keep the patient well filled

What is the management of flap venous congestion?

The flap is purple and oedematous with a brisk CRT
1. Elevate if possible
2. Inform the operating surgeon
3. Consider leech therapy and anticoagulation

If no action is taken, the flap is at risk of ischaemia due to the developing positive pressure gradient

PLASTIC SURGERY OF THE BREAST

BREAST ANATOMY

What is the arterial supply of the breast?

The pectoral branch of the thoracoacromial artery anastomoses with the internal mammary artery and the external mammary branch of the lateral thoracic artery to supply the breast. Perforating thoracic branches of the intercostals also contribute. A subdermal plexus supplies the skin

What is the venous drainage of the breast?

Circulus venosus is an anastomotic circle around the base of the nipple. Veins branch out radially from here and drain into the axillary and internal mammary veins

What is the lymphatic drainage of the breast?

Breast lymph drains mainly via axillary lymph nodes (from levels I to III), and partially to clavicular lymph nodes

How is the breast innervated?

With lots of overlap. Anterior and lateral branches of the 4th, 5th and 6th intercostal nerves provide innervation in a dermatomal fashion

The nipple lies in the dermatome of the 4th intercostal nerve which has a deep and superficial branch. The **deep branch** passes inferolaterally on the pectoralis major fascia then courses up to supply the areola. The **superficial branch** passes up through the superficial parenchyma

What are the relations of the breast?

The breast lies within the superficial fascia with the 2nd rib above and the 6th rib below. It extends medially from the lateral border of the sternum to the mid axillary line laterally

The **axillary tail** of the breast extends up into the base of the axilla

The breast is separated from pectoralis major and its investing fascia by a layer of loose connective tissue

What is the breast made of?

Glandular tissue embedded in fat with ducts converging on the nipple

BREAST AUGMENTATION

What are the indications for breast augmentation?

Aesthetic improvement of the dimensions and volume of breasts in a patient with *realistic* expectations

What are the specific contraindications?

Breast malignancy. Smoking worsens outcome

PART III

What are the elements of pre-op planning?

1. Informed consent
2. Implant options: implant size, textured versus smooth, anatomic (tear drop) versus round
3. Placement options: submuscular (implant under pectoralis major) versus subglandular (implant under glandular tissue of the breast)
4. Incision options: transaxillary, inframammary, periareolar or transumbilical
5. Consider a mammogram

Give a specific complication of augmentation?

Capsular contracture: an exaggerated scar **breast** response to the foreign material resulting in symptoms ranging from firm texture of the breast to distorted, hard, painful, cold breast

What is the incidence of this?

Up to 30%

How is it treated?

It can be managed surgically with capsulectomy, implant exchange or implant removal

What other complications do you know of?

1. Haematoma
2. Seroma
3. Wound infection
4. Altered nipple sensation
5. Mondor disease (superficial thrombophlebitis)
6. Implant problems: displacement, rippling, deflation or rupture (rare)

What is the post-op care following breast augmentation?

The patient can be discharged early with analgesia and prophylactic antibiotics (3–5 days). They should be advised against rigorous exercise for 2–3 weeks. Follow up should begin around 5 days after the procedure

BREAST REDUCTION

What are the indications for breast reduction?	Uncomfortably large breasts indicated by symptoms such as upper back pain, neck pain, shoulder pain and grooving from bra straps, breast pain and infra-mammary intertrigo
What are the specific contraindications?	Current lactation or recent lactation (within the last 9 months), malignancy or suspected malignancy
What is important in pre-op management?	Consider mammography if the patient is over 35 years old or has a high risk of developing breast cancer. Ensure patient has given informed consent
What types of breast reduction are there?	Many types. Decision based on the size of reduction, breast shape and surgeon preference **Options include**: inferior pedicle, central pedicle, lateral pedicle, bipedicle, medial pedicle and short scar techniques. Breast reduction can be liposuction-assisted
What are the specific complications of breast reduction?	1. Nipple loss or nipple–areolar complex loss are more common in smokers and patients who have had extremely large breasts 2. Skin necrosis 3. Fat necrosis 4. Asymmetry 5. Loss of sensation of the breast skin (uncommon)
What is the post-op care following breast reduction?	Early discharge with analgesia. Use of antibiotics and support garments depends on surgeon's preference. Rigorous exercise should be avoided for 2–3 weeks post-operatively

PART III

BREAST RECONSTRUCTION

What types of breast reconstruction are there?	Submuscular implant, expander implant and transposition flap reconstruction

What types of transposition flap reconstruction are there?

1. **Distant**: Rectus abdominus, latissimus dorsi
2. **Microvascular**:
   a. Rectus abdominus
   b. Deep inferior epigastric perforator (DIEP)
   c. Inferior gluteal perforator
   d. Gluteus maximus

What are the indications for flap reconstruction?

1. Post-mastectomy when there is inadequate local tissue for implant augmentation
2. Unacceptable overlying skin
3. Radiation damage

What are the contraindications?

Absolute:
1. Prior division of the flap muscle
2. Congenital absence of the flap muscle
3. Continuing active disease in lymph nodes
4. Metastases

Relative:
1. Smoking
2. Plans for adjuvant radiotherapy or prior irradiation
3. Prior division of the vessels supplying the flap

What is the pre and post-op management?

It follows the principles of flap management described earlier

CLEFT LIP AND CLEFT PALATE

What is cleft lip and cleft palate?	They are common congenital abnormalities resulting from failure of closure of either the primary or secondary palate, or both
What is the primary palate?	The primary palate consists of the following: 1. Pre-maxilla (anterior nasal spine and 4 incisor teeth) 2. Anterior septum 3. Soft tissues of the upper lip
What is the secondary palate?	The structures posterior to the incisive foramen, including the remains of the hard palate, soft palate and uvula
How can they become clefted independently?	Due to the separate embryogenesis of the lip and the palate. There are multiple classifications to describe the morphology of a cleft
What are the indications for repair?	Any cleft lip or palate can be repaired. The reasons are: 1. To achieve normal speech 2. To improve feeding and swallowing 3. Aesthetic reasons (cosmesis)
At what age is the operation carried out?	Repair can be a multistage undertaking. The primary corrective operation is usually performed when the infant is 10–12 months old (near the time of language acquisition)

What are the pre-op considerations?

Pre-clerking: full history and examination may reveal the presence of associated abnormalities requiring further investigation before an anaesthetic is given (cleft lip and palate may occur as part of congenital syndromes)

It should also include documentation of developmental status, and audiologic evaluation in the case of a cleft palate (ENT abnormalities may co-exist)

Imaging: specialist imaging may be required, eg 3D CT scan to assess bone deficiency

The patient should be measured and marked by the operating surgeon

What is the most dangerous complication of cleft lip and airway palate repair?

The complications are greater the more extensive the operation. The most dangerous is **obstruction**, especially if the operation has extensively involved the nose resulting in oedema or haematoma formation

Which population is this particularly dangerous in?

In infants, as they are obligate nasal breathers

What other complications are there?

1. Bleeding (may necessitate a return to theatre)
2. Infection
3. Wound disruption
4. Fistula formation
5. Ischaemic loss of the pro-labial flap
6. Hypertrophic scarring

CHAPTER 11: NEUROSURGERY

CLINICAL ANATOMY

What are the layers of the scalp?	*Mnemonic:* **SCALP** **S**kin **C**onnective tissue **A**poneurosis **L**oose connective tissue **P**eriosteum
What bones make up the skull?	Frontal, parietal, occipital, temporal, sphenoid, ethmoid, inferior nasal concha, lacrimal, vomer, nasal, zygomatic, maxilla, palatine, mandible Skull bones are joined at sutures and subdivided into **cranium** [vault (upper) and base of skull (lower)] and **facial skeleton**
Which bones make up the base of skull?	The following: 1. Roof of orbit (frontal bone) 2. Cribriform plate (ethmoid bone) 3. Sphenoid bone 4. Squamous and petrous parts of temporal bone 5. Occipital bones
What are the openings in the base of the skull and what structures pass through them?	See Table 11.1

Table 11.1

Cranial Fossa	*Opening*	Structures passing through
Anterior	Cribriform plate	CN I (olfactory n.)
Middle	Foramen ovale	CN V3 (mandibular division of trigeminal n) Lesser petrosal n.
	Foramen rotundum	CN V2 (maxillary division of trigeminal n.)
	Foramen spinosum	Middle meningeal a. and v.
	Foramen lacerum	Internal carotid a. Greater petrosal n.
	Optic canal	CN II (optic n.) Ophthalmic a.
	Superior orbital fissure	Frontal, lacrimal and nasociliary nn., all branches of CN V1 (ophthalmic branch of trigeminal n.) CN III (oculomotor n.), both branches CN IV (trochlear n.) CN VI (abducent n.) Superior ophthalmic v. Sympathetic nn.
Posterior	Foramen magnum	Medulla oblongata CN XI (spinal accessory n.) Vertebral aa.
	Hypoglossal canal	CN XII (hypoglossal n.)
	Internal acoustic meatus	CN VII (facial n.) CN VIII (vestibulocochlear nn.) Internal jugular vein (forms from sigmoid sinus)

How are structures passing through the superior orbital fissure remembered?	*Mnemonic:* **L**uscious **F**ried **T**omatoes **S**it **N**aked **I**n **A**nticipation **O**f **S**auce **L**acrimal n. **F**rontal n. **T**rochlear n. **S**uperior branch of oculomotor n. **N**asociliary **I**nferior branch of oculomotor n. **A**bducent n. **O**phthalmic vv. **S**ympathetic nn.
What are the anatomical divisions of the brain?	**Cerebral hemispheres** (frontal, parietal, temporal and occipital lobes) **Brainstem** (midbrain, pons, medulla) **Cerebellum**
What is its main blood supply?	As follows: • **Anterior circulation**: internal carotid artery (ICA) divides into anterior and middle cerebral aa. Mainly supplies frontal, temporal and parietal lobes as well as the deep grey matter • **Posterior circulation**: vertebral aa. join to form basilar a., which divides into 2 posterior cerebral aa. The vertebral a. also gives off the anterior spinal a. of the spinal cord and the posterior inferior cerebellar artery (PICA). The basilar a. gives off the anterior inferior cerebellar artery (AICA) and the superior cerebellar artery (SCA). Branches of basilar a. supply mainly the pons, cerebellum, thalamus and the posterior cerebral arteries supply the occipital lobes

What is the Circle of Willis?	An arterial anastomosis. The anterior communicating a. between the two anterior cerebral aa. and the two posterior communicating aa. between the internal carotid and posterior cerebral aa. form anastomoses between the anterior and posterior circulation as well as between the left and right systems
What is its venous drainage?	As follows: • **Superficial system**: superior sagittal sinus joins straight sinus, which forms transverse and sigmoid sinuses that exit the skull as the internal jugular vein (IJV). It drains the cortex and subcortical white matter • **Deep system**: the internal cerebral vv. and inferior sagittal sinus drain into straight sinus
What layers make up the meninges?	*Mnemonic:* The meninges **PAD** the brain **P**ia (innermost) **A**rachnoid (middle) **D**ura (outer): tough and thick, restricts the movement of the brain within the skull, which protects the brain from movements that may cause vascular damage
What are the names and functions of the twelve cranial nerves?	See Table 11.2

Table 11.2

Number	Name	Function	Supply
CN I	Olfactory	Smell	**Sensory**
CN II	Optic	Vision	**Sensory**
CN III	Oculomotor	Somatic motor supply to levator palpebrae superioris, superior, medial and inferior rectus muscles	**Motor**
		Parasympathetic supply to ciliary and papillary constrictor muscles	
CN IV	Trochlear	Somatic motor supply to superior oblique muscle	**Motor**
CN V	Trigeminal	Motor supply to muscles of mastication	**Both**
		Sensory supply to head and neck, sinuses, meninges and external surface of tympanic membrane	
CN VI	Abducens	Motor supply to lateral rectus muscle	**Motor**
CN VII	Facial	Motor supply to muscles of facial expression	**Both**
		Parasympathetic supply to glands of the head except the parotid, sensory supply to the ear and tympanic membrane	
		Taste to anterior two-thirds of tongue	
CN VIII	Vestibulocochlear	Hearing and balance	**Sensory**
CN IX	Glossopharyngeal	Motor supply to stylopharyngeus	**Both**
		Supplies parotid gland and carotid body	
CN X	Vagus	Motor supply to muscles of pharynx and larynx	**Both**
		Parasympathetic supply to neck, thorax and abdomen	
CN XI	Spinal accessory	Motor supply to trapezius and sternocleidomastoid muscles	**Motor**
CN XII	Hypoglossal	Motor supply to tongue muscles except palatoglossal	**Motor**

How are the cranial nn. supply remembered?

Mnemonic: **S**ome **S**ay **M**arry **M**oney, **B**ut **M**y **B**rother **S**ays **B**ig **B**reasts **M**atter **M**ore (in that order; see Table 11.2 above)

CNS TRAUMA AND INTRACRANIAL BLEEDS

What are the key abnormalities on scalp/occiput examination?

Remember: the more visible the injury, the more invisible (intracranial) injury may be present. Any lacerations should be cleaned, assessed and closed if possible.
Key points:

History
- Mechanism of injury (penetrating, missile, blunt trauma)
- Tetanus immunisation status
- Time elapsed since injury

Clean and explore
- Foreign bodies
- Dirt in wound
- Exploration to assess length and depth
- Boggy swelling suggesting underlying #

Is a skull X-ray indicated?
- High velocity injury
- Assault with a weapon
- Marked bruising or extensive laceration
- Any focal neurological deficit or drop in GCS

Is it an open #?
- Is there a bony # underneath the wound, implying direct contact between body surface and cranial vault?
- Requires neurosurgical consultation
- Take advice before closing
- May need IV antibiotics and continued observation

Can it be closed in the resus room?

- If deterioration demands transfer, control with pressure dressings is preferred to delay
- Scalp avulsions may require plastic surgery opinion
- Close with non adsorbable sutures if appropriate, or staples for speed

What is meant by 1ry and 2ry brain injury?

Primary brain injury: initial brain injury sustained at time of incident due to direct trauma/mechanical insult

Secondary brain injury: continuing damage to cerebral tissue caused by an altered chemical environment and/or impaired physiology; causes:

- Hypoxaemia
- Hypercarbia
- Hypotension

What intracranial lesions must be considered in a closed head injury (no laceration apparent)?

Skull #: suggested by high impact injury with boggy swelling at site

Basal skull #: suggested by the following signs

- Panda eyes
- Haemotympanum (blood behind the eardrum)
- CSF rhinorrhoea
- Battle's sign (mastoid bruising)

Extra-dural haematoma:

- Haematoma collecting between skull vault and dural layer of meninges
- Causes raised ICP and deteriorating neurological function
- Often caused by damage to the middle meningeal artery running through the temporal skull
- Often needs surgical evacuation via burr hole or craniotomy/bone flap

PART III

Subdural haematoma: haematoma under the dura but above the arachnoid layer, often caused by shearing of cortical draining veins

Subarachnoid haemorrhage/ intracerebral bleed: bleeding into the subarachnoid space/brain substance

Coup and contre-coup: as the brain is mobile in a fluid-filled cavity, rapid deceleration can cause injury/ contusion at the point of impact, with rebound injury at the opposite side

Diffuse axonal injury: may cause varying degrees of amnesia

What are the indications for a skull X-ray?

Considered when a CT head will not be performed, but concerns regarding skull fractures or intracranial trauma exist:

- High velocity injury
- Focal neurological signs
- Loss of consciousness or any alteration in conscious level post injury
- Marked superficial trauma

What are the indications for a CT scan of the head?

Immediate CT scanning is suggested in the following situations:

- Vomiting >2 episodes post head injury
- Focal neurological signs
- GCS <13 at any time since injury
- GCS 13/14 2 hours post injury
- Post traumatic seizure
- Any signs of a basal skull #/ open skull #
- Loss of consciousness or amnesia in patients >65 years or with any coagulopathy

CT scanning is also recommended within 8 hours for those patients with none of the above, but with a history of retrograde amnesia >30 min or loss of consciousness, with a dangerous mechanism of injury (RTA or fall >5 m)

What is the management of severe head injury?

In severe head injury either clinically or as picked up by CT scan, do the following:

- Intubation and ventilation
- Maintenance of normocarbia
- Prophylactic antibiotics for open/basal skull #
- IV mannitol to decrease ICP/steroids usually given on the advice of neurosurgical consult
- Urgent neurosurgical opinion

How is a patient with potential spinal injury immobilised?

1. Hard collar: prevents flexion/extension
2. Sandbags with in line stabilisation: prevents lateral flexion/rotation
3. Spinal board: used for extraction from hostile environment

How should a stabilised C-spine be approached?

Above all do no harm. Patients should remain in C-spine immobilisation until fully investigated and assessed:

History: including mechanism of injury, symptoms, previous injuries or operations on spine

Clinical exam

- Full PNS exam should be performed to evaluate potential uni/bilateral weakness, paraesthesia, hyperreflexia, hypertonia, and other signs suggestive of spinal cord injury

- With the C-spine manually immobilised by an assistant, the hard collar is removed and the spine palpated for any bony abnormalities (steps or swelling), subjective pain and tenderness. Spinal movements should not be evaluated here. Full spinal precautions should be replaced after the exam

What C-spine films would you order?

AP, lateral, and odontoid peg films

What *must* you be able to see on the lateral film?

Film *must* include C7/T1 junction. If this cannot be adequately obtained due to patient's condition, two options exist:
- Manual traction on the patient's arms inferiorly and repeat
- Swimmers view/trauma oblique – shoot through with shoulder abducted to 140°

What if this *still* doesn't work?

CT scan of the C-spine (often performed with the cranial scan)

VASCULAR NEUROSURGICAL CONDITIONS

SUBARACHNOID HAEMORRHAGES (SAH)

What is a SAH?

Bleeding into the subarachnoid space

What is the usual cause?

A burst aneurysm, most commonly a **Berry aneurysm** of the circle of Willis

What is the classical presentation of a SAH?

Pt. complains of 'worst headache of life', with nausea and vomiting, syncope, meningism (stiff neck), photophobia

If a SAH is suspected what is investigation of choice?

95% detected by CT brain. Angiography can determine the site of the bleeding aneurysm

When is a lumbar puncture done?	If CT scan is negative. LP is sensitive for a SAH. Traumatic LP will result in bloody CSF that clears with successive bottles; the CSF with SAH remains bloody throughout. Also, LP opening pressure is usually high with SAH
What is the management?	Once diagnosed observe BP and control with calcium channel blockers. Monitor ECG, and prescribe IV steroids (eg dexamethasone) and analgesia Clipping of the aneurysm may be attempted
What is the late complication of SAH?	Communicating hydrocephalus
What is a hydrocephalus?	Increased brain CSF. **Communicating hydrocephalus** occurs at the level of the arachnoid granulations and **non-communicating** occurs proximal to them
What types do you know of?	Congenital and acquired
Gives some causes of acquired hydrocephalus	Meningitis, obstructed CSF absorption due to intraventricular haemorrhage or neoplasia
How does a hydrocephalus present?	Headache, nausea and vomiting, papilloedema. Late signs are lethargy and diplopia
What is the treatment of hydrocephalus?	**Communicating**: lumbar puncture relieves pressure **Non-communicating**: ventricular drainage Chronic hydrocephalus may require a shunt to divert excess CSF, eg ventriculoperitoneal

NEUROVASCULAR MALFORMATIONS

What types of vascular malformations are relevant to the neurosurgeon?	1. Arteriovenous (AV) malformations (most common) 2. Venous and cavernous angiomas 3. Telangiectasias
How do AV malformations commonly present?	Haemorrhage and seizures. Headaches are uncommon
How are AV malformations treated?	Either by surgical excision or embolisation

CNS TUMOURS

How do brain tumours commonly present?	Headaches, seizures, abnormal neurological findings
What are the most common primary brain tumours in adults?	Astrocytomas and meningiomas
What are the most common primary brain tumours in children?	Astrocytomas and medulloblastomas
From which sites do tumours commonly metastasise to the brain?	1. Bronchus 2. Breast 3. Renal 4. Gastrointestinal 5. Melanoma
What is a false lateralising sign?	A sign resulting from the presence of a tumour but not due to direct infiltration or compression by the tumour. For example: lateral rectus nerve palsy causing diplopia secondary to brain herniation, a direct result of increased intracranial pressure due to increasing tumour size

BRAIN ABSCESS

Which bacteria are most common pathogens?	**Adults**: streptococcal **Kids**: Gram −ve organisms **In AIDS**: *Toxoplasma gondii* **Traumatic**: staphylococcal
What is the most common source?	Pulmonary infections
What are risk factors for developing brain abscesses?	1. Systemic infections (pyogenic metastasis) 2. Sinus infections 3. Ear infections (CSOM, mastoiditis) 4. Cranial trauma 5. Immunosuppression
How are brain abscesses treated?	**Medical**: extended course of IV antibiotics **Surgical**: if there is a mass effect or if the abscess approaches the ventricles putting the ventricle at risk of rupture, intervention is necessary (I&D via craniotomy)

PAEDIATRIC CONDITIONS

What is the most prevalent congenital neural malformation?	Spina bifida occulta
What is spina bifida?	The congenital absence of the posterior spinal vertebrae resulting in exposure of the spinal cord and its coverings. Two forms: **occulta** and **aperta.** Occulta has skin (± hairy tuft) overlying the defect. Aperta is an open defect. (Syn. **rachischisis**)
What are the symptoms?	Leg paralysis, incontinence, mental retardation and associated hydrocephalus
How is it diagnosed?	May be picked up on USS *in utero*. Amniotic fluid is rich in AFP

PART III

What is an encephalocele?   Neural tissue protruding through a cranial defect, most commonly occurring in the occipital region

What is a meningocele?   Cystic posterior midline mass covered with membrane or skin, contains CSF and meninges. Most common site is the lumbosacral region

CHAPTER 12: CARDIOTHORACIC SURGERY

RELEVANT TERMINOLOGY

What is the stroke volume (SV)?	The volume of blood pumped after systole
What is the cardiac output (CO)?	**Heart rate (HR)** × **SV**. Normally 5 l/min. Is the gold standard for measuring cardiovascular function
What is the cardiac index?	**CO/TBSA** (total body surface area). Takes account of the patient's size and is more informative
What is the mean arterial pressure (MAP)?	This is the average pressure within an artery over a complete cycle of one heartbeat **MAP = Diastolic BP + 1/3(Systolic–Diastolic BP)** It is used to monitor end-organ perfusion
What is Starling's law?	The contractility of the heart is a measure of the myocardial muscle fibre length at the end of diastole, ie the more stretched the ventricle, the higher the cardiac output. If it exceeds the fibre length, then the cardiac output decreases (Frank–Starling curve)
How do you increase CO?	Increase pre-load Inotropes to increase contractility Increase chronotropes

How do you monitor the CO?

1. **Swann–Ganz catheter**: a balloon floatation catheter with 4 lumens is passed through the IJV, right atrium (RA) and then right ventricle. Allowed to float through the pulmonary artery (PA) to 'wedge' into a terminal branch. This wedge pressure has a direct correlation to the left atrial (LA) pressure. Through thermodilution methods, the CO, systemic and pulmonary vascular resistance (SVR & PVR) is calculated

2. **Oesophageal Doppler**: an external Doppler probe inserted into the anesthetised patient's oesophagus. As the RA lies posterior to the oesophagus, the probe can estimate RA filling. By using the Doppler principle, the CO & SVR are calculated

Can cardiovascular function be measured non-invasively?

Yes. ECG, BP, urine output (measure of end-organ perfusion), central venous pressure (CVP)

What does the CVP measurement indicate?

This is a dynamic measurement via cannulation at the IJV or subclavian v. The response to a fluid bolus will indicate whether a patient has adequate intravascular volume (providing the right and left sides of the heart are reciprocal)

CARDIAC SURGERY

APPLIED ANATOMY

What is the blood supply of the heart?

The right and left coronary arteries originate from the ascending aortic sinus. The left coronary artery (LCA) from the left posterior aortic sinus and the right coronary artery (RCA) from the anterior aortic sinus

What does the LCA supply?

This is larger in calibre than the RCA and supplies the majority of the left atrium and ventricle as well as the interventricular septum

What are the branches of the LCA?

The left main stem continues as the left anterior descending but also gives branches to the diagonal and circumflex arteries

What does the RCA supply?

The right atrium and ventricle

What are the branches of the RCA?

Right posterior descending artery (in 30% of people) and the marginal branches

What does the term 'dominance' mean?

It describes the origin of the posterior descending artery where left dominance implies that the origin is the left coronary artery and occurs in 70% of the population

When does coronary blood flow take place?

During diastole, from the sinuses of Valsalva

What is the venous drainage of the heart?

These mostly drain via small veins into the right atrium. A small amount drains directly into the right ventricle

Where are the atrioventricular valves?

The mitral (bicuspid) valve separates the left atrium and ventricle, and the tricuspid valve separates the right. They are supported by the chordae tendinae

PART III

Why are diseases more commonly on the left than right valves?

The left side of the heart involves the mitral and aortic valves which are on a high pressure to maintain the systemic circulation. The tricuspid and pulmonary valves serve the pulmonary circulation under low pressures

CORONARY ARTERY DISEASE (CAD)

What is CAD?

The development of atherosclerotic plaque within the coronary arteries. With time the plaque increases in size impeding the vessel lumen. If the plaque ruptures, thrombus forms as a reactionary process and leads to occlusion of the coronary artery and results in ischaemia

What is the incidence in the UK?

About 2.7 million and remains the leading cause of death in the UK

What are the risk factors for?

1. Hypertension
2. Smoking
3. Diabetes
4. Hyperlipidaemia
5. Positive family history (affects <60 years old) Others include: male gender, physical inactivity and race (Asian subcontinent)

How does it present?

CAD is a progressive disease. Presentation is dependent on the **degree of stenosis** of the coronary artery. Initially patients develop worsening symptoms during exercise where cardiac output increases and hence myocardial demand. If the stenosis increases, symptoms are of chest pain, shortness of breath, nausea and vomiting and feeling hot and sweaty, as with an MI

How is it diagnosed?

1. History
2. Examination (full CVS exam!)
3. ECG (±stress testing and thallium scan)
4. CXR
5. TTE (trans-thoracic echocardiogram)
6. Coronary angiography

What are the ECG findings?

This can be done under stress (exercise tolerance) for symptoms of chest pain (**Bruce protocol**). The changes are of **heart strain** initially (ST depression), followed by ST elevation in an MI. The leads indicate different aspects of the heart:

Leads II, III, aVF	inferior aspect
Leads V1-V2	anterior aspect
Leads V3-V4	septum
Leads V5-V6	lateral aspect

What is a thallium scan?

Under continuous ECG and BP monitoring, the patient's heart is stressed with exercise. Radioactive Thallium-201 (a potassium analogue taken up by contracting myocardial cells) is injected and a camera is used to then detect areas of poor myocardial perfusion. It is then repeated at 2 and 4 hours

What are the CXR findings?

With long-term myocardial ischaemia, the patient may develop heart failure where demand exceeds supply. The heart dilates and fluid builds up in the lungs. The CXR findings are:

Mnemonic: **ABCDEF**

A – **A**lveolar shadowing
B – Air **B**ronchogram, Kerley **B** lines
C – **C**ardiomegaly
D – Upper lobe **D**iversion
E – Pleural **E**ffusions
F – **F**luid in the **f**issure

PART III

What are the TTE findings?	May show dyskinetic (non-moving) segments of the heart corresponding to a previous MI. It also indicates the competency of the aortic and mitral valves
What are the findings of angiography?	A catheter is inserted at the groin though the femoral artery and fed back into the coronary artery sinuses. A dye is injected and the patency of the vessels seen. The degree of coronary stenosis dictates the number of grafts
What is the treatment of CAD?	The aim is to: 1. Maintain coronary blood flow 2. Increasing CO **Medical**: nitrates (vasodilators), diuretics and antihypertensives (increase CO) **Minimally invasive**: percutaneous coronary angioplasty (PCA) ± stenting **Surgical**: coronary artery bypass surgery (CABG)

CORONARY ARTERY BYPASS SURGERY (CABG)

What is cardiopulmonary bypass (CPB)?	An integral part of open heart procedures (CABG, valve repair and replacements and transplant) to ensure that the heart and lung are bypassed and the heart remains still during grafting with no lasting effects of ischaemia
How is it performed?	A venous catheter is connected to the RA to remove the systemic venous blood to an external machine which filters, warms, oxygenates and filters the blood which is then returned in a **non-pulsatile manner** to another catheter connected to the ascending aorta

Why is anticoagulation necessary?

Heparin is given prior to CPB and during the procedure to prevent thrombosis in the machine. Following the procedure and removal of the catheters, **protamine** is administered to reverse the procedure

What is cardioplegia?

This is provided via a different catheter into the coronary circulation. It cools down the heart and decreases its metabolic rate. Together these reduce the electrical activity in the heart and make it motionless for surgery

What are the complications of CPB?

CVS: thrombocytopenia, arrhythmias
RS: pulmonary atelectasis (bi-basal collapse), pneumonia
GI: upper GI bleeding, pancreatitis, bowel ischaemia
CNS: stroke

What is done if a patient fails to come off CPB?

1. Inotropes
2. Intra-aortic balloon pump
3. External pacing

What is an intra-aortic balloon pump (IABP)?

It is a balloon placed in the aorta through the femoral a. It inflates in diastole increasing diastolic BP and improving myocardial blood flow. It deflates in systole and increases the systolic BP

What is CABG?

A surgical procedure which aims to bypass the stenosed segment of coronary a. by using the internal mammary a., a length of long saphenous v. or radial a. It may or may not use CPB

PART III

What are the indications for CABG?

1. Significant left main coronary stenosis
2. 70% stenosis of LAD
3. Triple vessel disease
4. Unstable angina/disabling angina despite maximal therapy

What layers do you go through to reach the heart?

1. Skin
2. Fat
3. Superficial and deep fascia
4. Periosteum
5. Sternum
6. Fibrous pericardium
7. Pericardial fluid (normally minimal unless recent MI, pericarditis or tamponade)
8. Heart (surrounded by visceral pericardium)

What are the steps of CABG?

1. Under GA, a median sternotomy is performed
2. Following anticoagulation with heparin, CPB and cardioplegia, the segment of saphenous vein or radial artery is anastomosed distal to the blocked branch of the coronary artery (bottom end), and then to the aorta (top end)
3. The patient is then re-warmed and taken off CPB
4. The chest is closed with sternal wires
5. Patient transferred to ITU

What are the complications of CABG?

Early:
1. Arrhythmia
2. Haemorrhage
3. Stroke
4. Pneumonia
5. MI/graft occlusion
Late: sternal dehiscence

What is the prognosis?

The mortality is 1% for elective CABG

What are the post-op medications?

1. Aspirin
2. Statin (eg simvastatin)
3. ACE inhibitor (if normal renal and liver function)
4. Beta-blockers if the patient was having pre-operatively

Which arrhythmia is most common post CABG?

Atrial fibrillation (AF) in up to a third of patients

How is AF managed post-op?

1. CXR and echo to exclude a pericardial collection
2. Correction of electrolytes (K and Mg)
3. Medical cardioversion (amiodarone and beta-blockers)
4. Direct current cardioversion if all else fails

How are arrhythmias managed intra-operatively?

If any arrhythmias are noted intra-op post bypass, the surgeon may insert some pacing wires into the atrium, ventricle or both

What are the modes of pacing?

These are usually represented in 3 letters, the 1st indicating the chamber paced, the 2nd indicating the chamber sensed and the 3rd indicating the response, eg AAI indicates that the atria are being sensed and paced with an inhibition of pacing if the heart contracts at that point. D indicates dual chamber

What are the new types of CABG?

MIDCAB (minimally invasive coronary artery bypass): a mini sternotomy to reduce chances of infection
OPCAB (off pump coronary artery bypass): grafting is done with no CPB to reduce risks of complications

PART III

VALVULAR HEART DISEASE (VHD)

What is VHD?

This is stenosis (narrowing), regurgitation (incomplete closure), or atresia (incomplete development from birth) of the atrioventricular (mitral and tricuspid), aortic or pulmonary valves

What is the aetiology of VHD?

1. Rheumatic fever
2. Senile calcification
3. Post-MI
4. Congenital
5. Severe lung disease
6. Bacterial endocarditis

What is rheumatic fever?

Predominantly a paediatric disease affecting joints, heart and skin secondary to infection by Group A haemolytic streptococcus. It causes a cross reaction of cardiac proteins resulting in thickening and stenosis of the heart valves

What are the symptoms of valve disease?

Can be symptomless early in the disease process. With time patients develop fatigue, palpitations, angina or symptoms of heart failure (exertional dyspnoea)

How is the severity of dyspnoea classified?

Into the New York Heart Association classification:

NYHA I	Capable of ordinary physical activity
NYHA II	Ordinary activity induces dyspnoea
NYHA III	Limitation of physical activity
NYHA IV	Symptoms at rest

How is it diagnosed?

A Doppler echocardiogram (trans-thoracic or trans-oesophageal) is the investigation of choice

What are the echo findings?

Combined with colour, Doppler may show regurgitation. Where stenosis is evident, the gradient across the valve increases

What is the treatment of VHD?

This depends on the type and severity of disease.

Medical therapy:

1. **ACE inhibitors**: to maintain a low BP and offload the heart
2. **Antiarrhythmics**: to prevent arrhythmias occurring with a dilated atrium
3. **Anticoagulants**: to avoid clots dislodging into the systemic circulation

What are the indications for surgery?

1. Worsening symptoms
2. Worsening ECG changes
3. Bacterial endocarditis refractive to medical therapy
4. Enlargement of the atrium on CXR/echo ± arrhythmias (for mitral valve disease)

What investigation is essential prior to surgery?

A coronary angiogram to check if there are any coronary vessels occluded. If so a combined procedure of CABG and valve repair/replacement is done

What are surgical options for VHD?

Percutaneous valvuloplasty: for mitral stenosis; a balloon catheter is passed to the valve and inflated

Valve repair/valvotomy: for mitral regurgitation; open procedure involving CPB, and may involve insertion of an annular ring to strengthen the chordae

Valve replacement: 2 types:

Mechanical (St Jude, Starr–Edwards): these may last a lifetime but require lifelong anticoagulation post-op due to the risk of thromboembolism

PART III

Xenografts (porcine, bovine, pericardial): these are less durable lasting 10–15 years. Anticoagulation is more controversial and tends to be short-lived for 3–6 months. Xenografts are reserved to the elderly population to avoid the risks of anticoagulation

What are the features of the main valvular disorders?

See Table 12.1

Table 12.1

	Aortic stenosis	Aortic regurgitation	Mitral stenosis	Mitral regurgitation
Definition	Narrowing of aortic valve opening. Either congenital with bicuspid valves, or 2ry to senile calcification or rheumatic fever (RhF)	Aortic valve leaflets do not close in diastole allowing backflow of blood into the left ventricle. Occurs with bacterial endocarditis (BE), RhF, connective tissue diseases (eg Marfan's)	Narrowing of mitral opening between the left atrium and ventricle. Occurs due to RhF, calcification. Occurs more in females (**Ms. = MS!**)	The 3 mitral valve leaflets do not oppose during ventricular systole allowing backflow of blood from the left ventricle. Occurs with RhF, post MI (ruptured chordae). Occurs more in males (**Mr. = MR!**)
Symptoms	Angina, syncope, exertional dyspnoea	Angina, palpitations, dyspnoea	Angina, dyspnoea and hoarseness (dilated atrium compresses on recurrent laryngeal nerve)	Palpitations, dyspnoea
Signs	Slow rising pulse, left ventricular heave, ejection systolic murmur	Collapsing pulse, displaced apex, early diastolic murmur, Corrigan's sign, pistol shot femoral	Malar flush, AF, mid-diastolic murmur	AF, heave, pansystolic murmur

Table 12.1 *Continued*

	Aortic stenosis	Aortic regurgitation	Mitral stenosis	Mitral regurgitation
Echo findings	Severe if gradient of more than 40 mmHg, valve area <0.5cm^2	Regurgitant flow	Significant if valve orifice <1 cm^2/m^2 body surface area	Regurgitant jet

CONGENITAL CARDIAC CONDITIONS

Which are the cyanotic heart diseases?

These cause mixing of oxygenated and de-oxygenated blood.
Mnemonic: they all begin with **T**
Tetralogy of Fallot
Transposition of the great vessels
Truncus arteriosus
Tricuspid atresia

Which are the acyanotic heart diseases?

Here the blood reaching the right side of the heart passes to the lungs via the pulmonary vasculature in a normal fashion. These are patent ductus arteriosus, coarctation of aorta, ASD, VSD. (See Table 12.2)

VENTRICULAR SEPTAL DEFECT (VSD)

When does the septum develop?

During heart development in the 1st 8 weeks of gestation. It forms from the downward growth of the septum primum and septum secundum to join the interventricular septum

What is a VSD?

The most common congenital heart defect where the interventricular septum does not fully form leaving a defect

How common is VSD?

1% of babies are born with a VSD, though the majority are too small to be symptomatic

What are the types of VSD?

Peri-membranous: more common (75% of cases) and occurs in the upper portion near the valves
Muscular: occurs in the lower segment of the septum (25% of cases)

What are the complications of a VSD?

Due to the increased pressures in the LV, anatomical left to right shunting of blood occurs leading to increased pulmonary blood flow and right ventricular hypertrophy. With time it leads to irreversible pulmonary hypertension and **right to left shunting (Eisenmenger's syndrome)**

What are the symptoms and signs of a VSD?

Occur mostly in childhood and depend on the size of the defect. They range from fatigue, sweating, dyspnoea, to failure to thrive. A pansystolic murmur is evident

How is it diagnosed?

Incidental murmur, leading to a TTE or TOE. Cardiac MRI is now used to delineate the anatomy of the VSD

What is the treatment?

Depends on the size and symptoms. If small and symptomless, the defect may close with age
Medical management: diuretics (to offload the right heart), antihypertensives and antiarrhythmics (digoxin)
Surgical management: closure of the VSD. Once Eisenmenger's syndrome has ensued, the only option is a heart/lung transplant

ATRIAL SEPTAL DEFECTS (ASD)

What is the incidence of ASD?

Around 4:100,000 live births

What are the causes of an ASD?

Like VSD, congenital closure of the septum primum and secundum is incomplete

What are the symptoms?

These present late. If the defect is small, patients may remain symptomless. With increasing size, symptoms include dyspnoea on exertion, palpitations, tiredness

How is it diagnosed?

Echocardiography (TTE or TOE) to reveal the size of the defect

How is it treated?

If a large defect is causing symptoms, intervention is necessary to close it **Percutaneously** via an **Amplatz device** or **surgically** by a midline sternotomy and closure with a pericardial/synthetic patch

What are the complications of ASD?

Pulmonary hypertension via left to right shunting (Eisenmenger's syndrome), arrhythmias, heart failure and bacterial endocarditis.

Do patients require prophylactic antibiotics?

Yes, for both ASDs and VSDs as the risk of bacterial endocarditis is greater

What is Ebstein's anomaly?

Congenital downward displacement of the tricuspid valve into the right ventricle. It is often associated with an ASD

Give some characteristics of some of the more common congenital heart disorders.

See Table 12.2

PART III

Table 12.2

	Patent ductus arteriosus	Tetralogy of Fallot	Coarctation of the aorta	Transposition of the great vessels
Definition	The ductus arteriosus connecting the pulmonary artery to the aorta fails to obliterate after birth and causes physiologic right-to-left shunting. It occurs due to hypoxia, hyperprostaglandinaemia	A combination of: 1. Overriding aorta 2. Right ventricular hypertrophy 3. Pulmonary stenosis 4. VSD	Narrowing of the thoracic aorta near the ligamentum arteriosum. Collateral circulation occurs via subclavian to IMA to intercostals to descending aorta	The aorta originates from the right ventricle and the pulmonary artery from the left ventricle. Is fatal if no septal defect is present for communication
Symptoms	Asymptomatic, failure to thrive, respiratory distress	'Blue' babies, fainting and tiredness with minimal effort	Headache, fatigue, lower limb claudication	Cyanosis and signs of heart failure
Signs	Acyanotic, 'grumbling' murmur	Cyanosis, clubbing, ejection murmur	Systolic murmur, BP difference in both arms, HTN	
Investigations	Echocardiogram	Cardiac catheterisation	CXR, echo-cardiogram, angiography	Cardiac catheterisation
Treatment	**Medical:** Prostaglandin inhibitors (*indomethacin*) **Surgical:** Ligation of the DA at 2 years of age	**Surgical:** 2 stage-1st stage **Blalock-Taussig shunt**, second stage complete repair	**Surgery:** Resection with end- to end anastomosis. If large defect, insertion of an interpositional Dacron graft	**Surgical:** arterial switch

HEART AND LUNG TRANSPLANT

Where is this procedure done?

In a specialised tertiary centre. A full multidisciplinary team is involved, including the patient and family, cardiothoracic surgeons, respiratory physicians, cardiologists, radiologists, nurses, physiotherapists and cardiac and respiratory technicians

What are the indications for heart/lung transplant?

1. In end-stage disease of the heart and lung
2. Complex congenital heart defects not amenable to surgical repair
3. Patients with Eisenmenger's syndrome
4. Patients with irreversible right heart failure and pulmonary hypertension

Who gets it?

No limitations in lower age limit, although dependent on donor size. The upper age limit is 60 years and depends on the physiological status of the patient. No sex preference

What are the pre-op investigations?

1. Routine blood investigations (FBC, renal, liver and bone profile, inflammatory markers)
2. CT scan (to assess thoracic size for donor matching and to check for other pathological conditions)
3. Echocardiogram
4. Lung function tests

Who are the donors?

Any consenting patient who has been pronounced brain dead (following brainstem examination). They are maintained on a ventilator. The organs are harvested and transported within 6 hours to the recipient, or else lungs develop irreversible injury

PART III

What are the donor's criteria?	1. Free of cardiopulmonary disease 2. Age less than 50 years 3. Clear lung fields on CXR 4. Maintaining oxygen saturations of 100% on 40% inspired oxygen
What are the relevant steps?	Following a median sternotomy, the procedure continues with the patient in CPB. The heart and lung are removed and the donor organs inserted
In which order are the organs anastomosed?	Trachea, then right atrium followed by the aorta
What post-op medications are essential?	Immunosuppressants. Patients are followed up every 2–4 weeks initially to assess for signs of organ rejection

THORACIC AORTIC DISSECTION

What is an aortic dissection?	A longitudinal split in the tunica media of the aorta. When the tunica intima tears, a false lumen forms for blood to pass through
Where does it originate?	3 classic anatomical locations: 1. Aortic root 2. 2 cm above the aortic root 3. Just distal to the left subclavian artery
What are the risk factors?	*Mnemonic:* **ABC** **A**therosclerosis/**A**neurysm/**A**rteritis **B**lood pressure (high) **C**onnective tissue disorders (eg Marfans, Ehlers–Danlos syndromes)
What is the epidemiology ?	Peaks in 40–60 year olds, M:F = 3:1, commoner in Afro-Caribbean populations

What are the clinical features?	Sudden-onset severe chest pain radiating to the back (classically between the shoulder blades), syncope and dyspnoea
What are the classifications?	**DeBakey classification**:

DeBakey classification:

Type I	The entire aorta is involved
Type II	Only the ascending aorta is involved
Type III	Only the descending aorta is involved

Stanford classification:

Type A	The ascending aorta is involved
Type B	The descending aorta is involved

What investigations are diagnostic?

1. CXR (widened mediastinum)
2. Spiral CT scan of thorax
3. Echocardiography

What is the treatment of ascending dissection?

This is DeBakey Type I and II or Stanford Type A. Treatment is **surgical** due to the risk of aortic incompetence, tamponade, aortic rupture. If the coronaries dissect, patients develop an MI

What is the treatment of descending dissection?

This is DeBakey Type III and IV or Stanford Type B
Medical: antihypertensives (beta-blockers)

What is an Edwards procedure?

In ascending dissections involving the sinus and aortic valve, a transposition graft to replace the ascending aorta, aortic valve replacement and re-implantation of the coronary arteries

THORACIC SURGERY

MEDIASTINAL MASSES

APPLIED ANATOMY

What is the mediastinum?

The virtual space between both pleural in the thoracic cavity

What are its borders?

Superiorly the thoracic inlet, laterally both pleura, inferiorly the diaphragm, anteriorly the sternum and posteriorly the thoracic vertebrae 1–12
(See figure below)

Figure 12.1

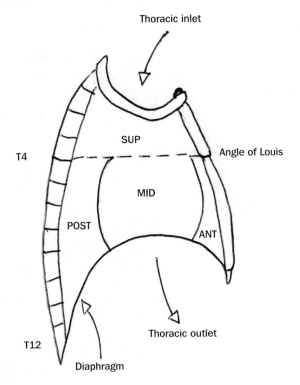

What are its divisions?

Superior and inferior mediastinum, divided by an imaginary transverse line from the manubriosternal junction anteriorly (**Angle of Louis**) and T4 posteriorly. The superior mediastinum has no divisions but the inferior mediastinum is further divided into the anterior, middle and posterior mediastinum

What are the contents of the superior mediastinum?

1. Thyroid gland
2. Aortic arch and great vessels
3. Oesophagus
4. Trachea
5. Vagus, recurrent laryngeal and phrenic nn.

And the anterior mediastinum?

1. Thymus gland
2. Lymph nodes
3. Internal mammary artery and vein
4. Fat and connective tissue

And the middle mediastinum?

1. Heart
2. Pulmonary arteries and veins
3. SVC and IVC

And the posterior mediastinum?

1. Oesophagus
2. Descending thoracic aorta
3. Azygos and hemiazygos vv.
4. Vagus and recurrent laryngeal nn.

What goes through the diaphragmatic openings?

There are 3 diaphragmatic apertures:
1. **The caval opening** (at T8): the IVC and phrenic nerve
2. **The oesophageal hiatus** (at T10): the oesophagus and vagal trunks
3. **The aortic hiatus** (at T12): the descending thoracic aorta (becomes abdominal aorta thereafter), azygos vein and thoracic duct

PART III

CLINICAL CONSIDERATIONS

What symptoms do patients experience?

May be asymptomatic

Specific compressive symptoms such as hoarseness (recurrent laryngeal nerve), dyspnoea (trachea), dysphagia (oesophagus), cough and SVC compression may occur

General symptoms include loss of weight and malaise

Tell me about some common mediastinal tumours

See Table 12.3

Table 12.3

	Content	Tumour/ Pathology	Diagnostic investigation	Characteristics	Treatment
Anterior mediastinum	Thymus gland	Thymoma	CT scan	Commonest tumour of the thymus and epithelial. M=F, occurs in the 5th to 7th decade. 25% are malignant	**Surgical resection.** Malignancy is noted intra-operatively with invasion into surrounding structures
	Thyroid gland	Papillary, follicular, medullary, anaplastic	USS/FNA	Depends on sub-type (see Chapter 11)	**Surgical:** Lobectomy vs total thyroidectomy
	Lymph nodes	Lymphoma	CXR/CT scan/ mediastinoscopy and biopsy	50% involve mediastinal nodes. Hodgkin's most common in mediastinum	**Non surgical:** Chemotherapy ± dexamethasone
	Fat/ connective tissue	Lipoma	CT/excisional biopsy	Benign, slow growing tumour of lipocytes	**Surgical excision** if causing compressive symptoms
		Teratoma	CXR/CT scan/ mediastinoscopy	Germ cell tumour from ectoderm, endoderm and mesoderm. (A dermoid cyst is ectodermal and contains teeth skin, hair). M=F, occurs in teenage years. 15% are malignant	**Surgical excision** after chemotherapy if malignant. 80% 5 year survival

Table 12.3 *Continued*

	Content	Tumour/ Pathology	Diagnostic investigation	Characteristics	Treatment
Middle mediastinum	Lymph-adenopathy	Lymphoma /sarcoid	CXR/CT/Bx		**Surgical excision**
	Heart	Atrial myxoma	Echocardiogram	Rare, benign tumour Patients may develop AF	**Surgical excision**
Posterior mediastinum	Oesophagus	Oeso-phageal tumour	CT scan	Squamous in most of oesophagus, adenocarcinoma at the gastro-oesophageal junction	(See below)
	Descending aorta	Aneurysm of the descending thoracic aorta	CT scan	Due to atherosclerosis and can lead to dissection	**Surgical replacement** with synthetic graft
	Nerves: sympathetic chain, vagus, recurrent laryngeal and phrenic			Commonest of mediastinal masses (20%–40%). Can arise from peripheral nerves (schwannoma, neurofibroma) or autonomic ganglia (ganglioneuroma, neuroblastoma)	**Surgical excision**

OESOPHAGEAL TUMOURS

What is the epidemiology of oesophageal tumours?

5th most common tumour in UK Incidence is 10:100,000. M:F = 2:1 Highest numbers in China, Japan

What are the risk factors?

Smoking, diet, excess alcohol, Barrett's oesophagus

What are the types of oesophageal tumours?

Squamous cell carcinoma in the upper ⅔ and adenocarcinoma in the distal ⅓ near the gastro-oesophageal junction 20% of all tumours occur in the upper part, 50% in the middle and 30% in the lower oesophagus

What are symptoms?

Dysphagia, weight loss, retrosternal chest pain and hoarseness with compression of the recurrent laryngeal nerve

What are the investigations?	1. Barium/gastrografin swallow
	2. OGD ± biopsies for the primary tumour
	3. CT chest and abdomen to detect extent and spread of tumour

What staging is advised?

The TNM (Tumour, Nodes, Metastases) staging is used, where **I and IIa** do not involve lymph nodes (80% 5-year mortality), **IIb and III** involve lymph nodes (20%–35% 5-year mortality) and **IV** involves distal metastases (0%–15% 5-year mortality)

What is an Ivor–Lewis operation?

A 2-step operation used for mid-oesophageal carcinoma. The 1st step is a **laparotomy** to mobilise the stomach. The 2nd step is a **lateral thoracotomy** at the 5th rib involving oesophageal resection and re-construction using the pulled-up stomach as an oesophageal substitute

What is mediastinitis?

This is inflammation of the mediastinum secondary to suppurative infection. It is caused by:
1. Oesophageal perforation/rupture (**Boerhaave's syndrome**) 2ry to excess vomiting or swallowed FB
2. Post-op sternal wound infection
3. Pneumonia or pleural infection
4. Distant infections and head and neck infections tracking down the pretracheal fascia

What is the prognosis?

It is a life-threatening condition with a 12%–45% mortality. Treatment is as with any emergency: A,B,C and IV antibiotics. The primary cause is then found and rectified

PLEURAL DISEASE

APPLIED ANATOMY

How many layers of pleura are there?

Two, the outer parietal layer is attached to the chest wall and the inner visceral layer attached to the lungs. The parietal pleura around the mediastinum is known as the mediastinal pleura

What is pleural fluid?

A serous lining secreted by the pleural mesothelium into the potential space between both layers of pleura. It allows lubrication during respiration

PLEURAL EFFUSION

What is a pleural effusion?

Fluid in the pleural space. Depending on protein content, it can be divided into exudative (>30 g/l) and transudative (<30 g/l)

What are the causes?

Exudates: an increased capillary permeability in the pleura secondary to **infection** (pneumonia, TB), **inflammation** (RA) or **malignancy** (bronchogenic carcinoma, metastases, mesothelioma, lymphoma)

Transudates: occur 2ry to increased venous pressure failure of heart, liver or kidneys

What are the symptoms?

May be asymptomatic, or c/o pleuritic chest pain, shortness of breath and/or decreased exercise tolerance

What are the signs?

Decreased expansion and breath sounds, and chest stony dull to percussion. Tracheal deviation if a large effusion present

PART III

What are the investigations?

1. CXR for diagnosis (look for blunting of the costophrenic angle in small effusions)
2. USS to confirm the presence and can guide accurate aspiration
3. Thoracentesis (needle drainage) can be therapeutic and diagnostic when fluid is sent for biochemistry, microbiology and cytology

If no cause is found, a **pleural biopsy** is taken surgically for histology (either thoracoscopic or open procedure through a mini thoracotomy)

What is the management?

Treat underlying cause. The treatment for the effusion is:

Chest drainage: via pigtail catheter or formal chest drain

Pleurodesis: if recurrent. This is an open or thoracoscopic procedure for draining the fluid and 'sticking' the 2 layers of pleura with talc (hence obliterating the potential space for future fluid collection). It is *not* done if the diagnosis is mesothelioma

Pleurectomy: if the above fail, the parietal pleura is stripped by either thoracoscopic or thoracotomy. The visceral pleura is sometimes abrased to allow an inflammatory process and hence adheres to the chest wall

What is a decortication?

This is done through thoracotomy for empyema (a collection of pus in the pleural cavity, mostly post pneumonic). A thick fibrous cortex originates from the empyema and surrounds the lung preventing expansion. This is removed surgically (**decortication**)

How do you insert a chest drain?

This is done under aseptic conditions. The area is previously marked from a recent CXR or USS

1. Local anaesthetic is applied to the pre-marked area (usually 5th intercostal space, anterior axillary line)
2. A green needle is passed to aspirate and ensure the presence of an effusion
3. A small skin incision is made just above the corresponding rib
4. Now blunt dissection only until the rib is reached and continue ABOVE the rib to avoid the intercostal's neurovascular bundle
5. Once the pleura is breached, the chest drain is guided using a long clip
6. The chest drain is now stitched in place and a purse-string suture applied. It is connected to an under-water seal to maintain a negative pressure
7. A post procedure CXR is essential to check positioning and for undue complications (pneumothorax)

PNEUMOTHORAX

What is a pneumothorax?

The presence of air within the pleural space. It occurs due to disruption of the parietal, visceral or mediastinal pleura. If the pleura forms a one-way valve, a **tension pneumothorax** forms and is a medical emergency

What are the different types of pneumothorax?

Three main types:
1. Spontaneous pneumothorax-
   a. **Primary**: in 85% of patients, no known cause is identified
   b. **Secondary**: in 15% of patients, an underlying pulmonary pathology is found
2. Traumatic pneumothorax: from blunt or penetrating thoracic trauma, or iatrogenic (post operative, post-CVP line insertion)

Who gets 1ry pneumothorax?

Occurs in young, slim tall men in their 20s to 30s M:F = 6:1. 10% are bilateral

What is the pathology behind it?

A congenital subpleural bulae which ruptures

What is the pathology of 2ry pneumothorax?

COPD, asthma, TB, pneumonia, lung cancer, cystic fibrosis, connective tissue disorders (eg Marfan's)

How is the diagnosis made?

CXR

What is the treatment?

A chest drain. The drain is positioned superiorly and an underwater seal connected. Bubbles indicate an ongoing defect. A swing in the drain indicates it is in the pleural space

What is the surgical treatment?

A talc pleurodesis (either thoracoscopic or via thoracotomy)

What is a haemothorax?

Blood in the pleural space. This may be 2ry to bronchitis, tumours, traumatic or iatrogenic (following chest drain insertion). If more than 700 ml/24 h is drained, it is termed a **massive haemothorax.** Treatment is ABCs, bronchoscopy ± surgical exploration

What is a chylothorax?

Lymphatic fluid in the pleural space 2ry to leakage from the thoracic duct. Causes are traumatic (and iatrogenic) and secondary to lymphoma. Treatment is via a chest drain or, if more than 1 l/day, surgery

MESOTHELIOMA

What is mesothelioma?

A tumour of the mesothelial cells which affects the pleura primarily (may rarely affect the peritoneum or pericardium)

What is its incidence?

1:1000,000, but the numbers are increasing fast

Who gets it?

M:F = 3:1. Patients are in the 4th to 6th decade (35 years following exposure to asbestos)

What is the cause?

Exposure to asbestos (occupational hazard in shipping yards, mines and mills)
Smoking

Is it benign or malignant?

It is highly malignant when diffuse. A localised mesothelioma may be benign but can also turn malignant

Where does it metastasise to?

Pulmonary parenchyma, chest wall, mediastinum, oesophagus and brachial plexus

What are the clinical features?

Pleuritic chest pain, dyspnoea, weight loss, clubbing, recurrent pleural effusions

What are the investigations?

1. CXR
2. CT scan thorax
3. Aspiration of pleural fluid for cytology
4. Pleural biopsy for histological analysis

PART III

What is the treatment?	Multi-modal therapy with surgical resection, chemotherapy and radiotherapy
What is the prognosis?	Very poor, with a survival after diagnosis of 1 year

LUNG CANCER

APPLIED ANATOMY

At what point does the trachea divide?	It divides into the right and left main bronchi at the level of T3/4. This is known as the **carina**
Where are foreign bodies most likely to lodge?	The right lower lobe for 3 reasons: 1. The right main bronchus has a wider lumen than the left as it delivers air to the bigger lung 2. The left main bronchus has a more acute angle to the left after bifurcation as it lies under the arch of aorta 3. The carina lies slightly to the left
What are the bronchial divisions?	The main (primary) bronchi divide into the lobar (secondary) bronchi, which further subdivide into the segmental (tertiary) bronchi. These supply the bronchopulmonary segments in each lung
What are the divisions of each lung?	The **right lung** has 3 lobes, the superior, middle and inferior. These are further subdivided into 10 bronchopulmonary segments The **left lung** has 2 lobes, the superior and inferior. The lingual is the remnant of the left middle lobe. It has 8–10 bronchopulmonary segments
Where do vessels and bronchi enter the lung?	At the hilum

CLINICAL CONSIDERATIONS

What is lung cancer?

A primary neoplasm of the lung

What is the incidence?

It is the most common cause of cancer deaths in men and second only to breast cancer in women. Causes 230:100,000 deaths

Who gets it?

M:F = 3:2, peaks at ages 65–75

What are the causes?

1. Cigarette smoking (except adenocarcinoma)
2. Asbestos exposure
3. Radon exposure

What are the histological types?

1. **Squamous cell carcinoma**: 50% of lung cancers; occurs in larger bronchi. Spreads to brain and bone
2. **Adenocarcinoma**: 5%–15% of lung cancers. Located peripherally. Metastasises to distant sites (adrenals, brain, bone, liver)
3. **Small cell (Oat cell) carcinoma**: 20% of lung cancers. 15% of patients have paraneoplastic syndromes. Disseminated, highly malignant and inoperable

What are the clinical features?

1. Chronic dry cough ±haemoptysis
2. Chest pain, dyspnoea
3. Hoarseness (if recurrent laryngeal nerve involvement)
4. Loss of power in the ipsilateral arm
5. Horner's syndrome (if invades the brachial plexus and sympathetic ganglia as in a Pancoast tumour)
6. Paraneoplastic syndromes (mostly in small cell tumours)
7. Finger clubbing

PART III

What are the pre-op investigation?

1. CXR (for obvious tumours)
2. Arterial blood gasses
3. Lung function tests
4. Flexible or rigid bronchoscopy
5. CT scan
6. PET scan

What is a PET scan?

Positron emission tomography. It administers a glucose analogue, fluorodeoxyglucose (FDG), to locate tumour metastases. Glucose is taken up by tumour cells at a higher rate, hence exposing them

What is the TNM staging of non small cell lung cancer?

Tumour (T)
T_1 <3 cm within the lung
T_2 >3 cm with pleural involvement
T_3 with extrapulmonary extension
T_4 involving the great vessels
Nodes (N)
N_0 No nodal involvement
N_1 Ipsilateral LN involvement
N_2 Contralateral LN involvement
Metastases (M)
M_0 No metastases
M_1 Distant metastases

What is the treatment and prognosis of the different stages?

See Table 12.4

Table 12.4

Stage	TNM	Description	Treatment	Prognosis (5 year survival)
I	T_1 or T_2 N_1 M_0	Any tumour size, with no extra pulmonary LN, no metastases	Surgical resection (lobectomy or pneumonectomy)	60%–85%
II	T_1 or T_2 N_2 M_0	Stage I tumour with positive LN in ipsilateral hilum, no metastases	Surgical resection	45%
IIIa	T_3 N_2 M_0	Any tumour size with extension to the pericardium, diaphragm or chest wall, but not great vessels. Ipsilateral LN involvement. No metastases	Surgical resection, chemotherapy, radiotherapy	30%
IIIb	T_4 N_3 M_0	Tumour extending to great vessels, contralateral LN involved. No distant metastases	Chemotherapy, Radiotherapy	10%
IV	M_1	Distant metastases	Chemotherapy	0%

What are the types of surgery?

A **lobectomy** vs **pneumonectomy**.
A lobectomy is advised if the tumour does not breach that particular pulmonary lobe
If the tumour is at the hilum involving 2 or 3 lobes, a pneumonectomy is advised providing the patient's lung function tests are good pre-operatively

What are the contraindications of surgery?

1. Patient co-morbidity
2. Small cell cancer (treated with chemo)
3. $FEV_1 < 1$
4. Carinal tumour involvement
5. Metastatic spread, (including supraclavicular LN)

CHAPTER 13: MAXILLOFACIAL SURGERY

NB Dental aspects of maxillofacial surgery have been omitted here. For details of these aspects, refer to a textbook of dentistry

FRACTURES

MANDIBULAR

What are mandibular #s claim to fame?	Most common # of the facial skeleton
How are they sustained?	Most are as a result of fights or RTA
Which part of the mandible is most commonly #d?	The mandibular condyle
How are mandibular #s classified?	As follows: 1. Dentoalveolar 2. Condyle 3. Coronoid 4. Ramus 5. Angle 6. Body
How is a mandibular # diagnosed?	1. History of trauma 2. Deranged occlusion 3. Sublingual haematoma 4. Bruising or swelling of face 5. Mobility of fragments 6. Bleeding (usually intra-orally) 7. Paraesthesia or anaesthesia of nerves involved in # site
Which X-rays are taken?	1. Orthopantogram (OPG) 2. PA mandible 3. Right and left lateral obliques (if OPG unobtainable) 4. Reverse Townes view (for condyles)
What are the most common radiological features?	1. Fracture lines 2. Step deformities 3. Widening of periodontal space (if teeth are involved)

How are mandibular #s managed?

Undisplaced #s may be managed conservatively with a soft diet
Displaced #s are managed by open reduction and fixation (ORIF) ± intermaxillary fixation (IMF)

MAXILLARY

How are maxillary #s classified?

By using the **Le Fort classification**:
Le Fort I: high level
Le Fort II: pyramidal
Le Fort III: low level or Guérin's #
(see Figure 13.1)

Figure 13.1

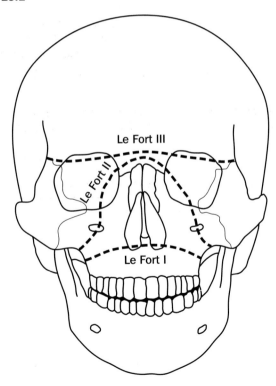

How are maxillary #s diagnosed?

1. History of *severe* trauma
2. Swelling: upper lip in Le Fort I #s; massive swelling of face and bilateral black eyes in severe Le Fort II and III #s (panda facies)
3. Pain
4. Bleeding (usually from nose), haematoma
5. Mobility, sometimes gross (floating face)
6. Posterior gagging of occlusion
7. Subconjunctival ecchymoses
8. Anaesthesia of the infraorbital nerves
9. Diplopia
10. Cerebrospinal rhinorrhoea (leakage of CSF through nose 2ry to disrupted cribriform plate)

Which X-rays should be taken?

Occipito-mental views 10° and 30°

How are maxillary #s managed?

Nearly all fractures are treated with ORIF with bone plates to reduce and fix all fragments accurately.
Occasionally a place for simple IMF

ORAL MANIFESTATION OF SYSTEMIC DISEASE

How may systemic disease manifest itself orally?

See Table 13.1

Table 13.1

System	Disease	Oral manifestation
Gastrointestinal	Coeliac disease Crohn's disease Cirrhosis Ulcerative colitis	Oral ulceration Linear long ulcers Granulations Purple swellings of lips, gingivae and buccal mucosa Glossitis (50% of patients) Oral ulceration
Endocrine	Acromegaly Addison's disease Cushing's syndrome Hypothyroidism Hyperparathyroidism Diabetes	Enlargement of tongue and lips Spacing of teeth Increase in jaw size Melanotic hyperpigmentation of oral mucosa 'Moon face' appearance Oral candidiasis Enlargement of the tongue Puffy enlarged lips Delayed tooth eruption Loss of lamina dura Ground glass appearance of bone Xerostomia and thirst Sialosis Burning mouth Oral and facial dysthesia

Table 13.1 *Continued*

System	Disease	Oral manifestation
Haematological diseases	Anaemia	Recurrent oral ulceration Atrophic glossitis Red beefy tongue Candidiasis Angular cheilitis Burning tongue
	Leukaemia	Painful oral lesions Increases tendency to bleed
	Cyclical neutropenia	Acute exacerbations of periodontal disease Candidiasis
	HIV/AIDS	Hairy leukoplakia Kaposi's sarcoma HIV periodontitis Acute ulcerative gingivitis
Skin diseases	Lichen planus	White reticular striae Erosive oral lesions
Connective disease	Ehlers–Danlos syndrome Rheumatoid arthritis	Pulp stones Hypermobility of the TMJ Sjögren's syndrome Rheumatoid of the TMJ (10%)

CHEILITIS

What is angular cheilitis?	Redness, soreness and ulceration usually affecting one or both angles of the mouth. Usually caused by staphylococcal infection, occasionally haemolytic streptococci
What is its aetiology?	1. Poorly fitting dentures 2. General ill health 3. Obscure anatomical features 4. Accompanies xerostomia 5. May be an early marker for AIDS 6. Poor oral hygiene 7. Steroid use

How is it managed?	1. Full history of complaint
	2. Topical antimicrobial
	3. Eliminate source of infection
	4. Remove predisposing factors

RECURRENT APHTHOUS ULCERATION

How common is recurrent aphthous ulceration (RAU)?

Approximately one in five of the population suffer from RAU at some time

What are the different types of RAU?

Minor, major and herpetic oral aphthae. (See Table 13.2)

Table 13.2

Oral aphthae	Minor	Major	Herpetic
% of RAU	80%	10%	10%
Size	2–4 mm	>1 cm	Multiple small ulcers
Sites affected	Non-keratinised sites	Posterior parts of mouth and keratinised sites	
Time taken for healing	3 weeks	Several weeks Leaves scarring	3 weeks

What is the aetiology?

1. Psychological (stress)
2. Trauma
3. Deficiency (iron, folic acid, vitamin B_{12})
4. Endocrine
5. Allergy
6. Smoking
7. Heredity

How are RAU managed?

Initial visit:
1. Full history of complaint
2. Chlorhexidine mouthwash
3. Dietary advice to avoid chocolate, benzoates

Review after 1 week:
If no improvement:
1. Hydrocortisone 2.5-mg pellet allowed to dissolve near ulcer qds
2. Triamcinolone paste, thin layer applied 2–4 times daily

ORAL CANCER

What is the incidence of oral carcinoma?

Accounts for approx 2% of all tumours in UK and USA, and approx 40% of tumours in India/Sri Lanka

What is the reason for this discrepancy in incidence?

The popularity of chewing **betel nut** in the Indian subcontinent. Betel nut is carcinogenic

What type of cancer is it?

Over 90% are squamous cell carcinomas

Who gets it?

98% of patients are over the age of 40
M:F = 3:2

What are the risk factors?

1. Excessive alcohol and smoking
2. Tobacco and betel nut chewing
3. Sunlight (lip only)
4. Mucosal diseases (lichen planus, oral submucous fibrosis, dysplastic lesions)
5. Infections (syphilis, candidiasis, viruses)
6. Genetic disorders (eg Fanconi's anaemia)

Where is the most common site of occurrence in the mouth?

70% form on the lateral borders of the tongue, adjacent alveolar ridge and floor of mouth

How would you recognise oral carcinoma?

Early stages:
1. Painless red, speckled patch
2. Erythroplakia
3. Non-healing ulcer

Late stages:
1. Painful ulcer, firm with raised edges, and an indurated, inflamed, granular base, fixed to surrounding tissues
2. Referred otalgia

How is the tumour staged?

The TMN staging is commonly used:
T primary tumour
T1 < 2 cm diameter
T2 2–4 cm diameter
T3 >4 cm diameter
T4 massive, invading beyond mouth
N cervical nodes
N0 no nodes
N1 single node <3 cm
N2 multiple ipsilateral nodes or single node 3–6 cm
N3 bilateral cervical nodes or ipsilateral node >6 cm
M distant metastases
M1 absent
M2 present

How does the tumour spread?

Spread is by direct invasion of surrounding tissues and by lymphatic metastasis. **Submandibular** and **jugulodiagastric** nodes are most frequently involved

How is oral carcinoma managed?

Depends on age and medical condition of pt., exact site and histological type. Treatment may be by surgery or radiotherapy

What is the 5-year survival rate?

90% for T1 N0; 30% for T2/3 N1. Worse for T4

INDEX

Page numbers followed by *g* indicate an entry in the Glossary. Page numbers in *italic* indicate a Table or illustration.

Lect.
1 — Copy Notes
2 — Write do notes for MB anatomy.
3 — Read Ethics
4 — Return Lib books
    Uni brm
5 — Sort out bills & accounts
6 — Tot out the amount harshv
    owes you.
7 — Locker key —